This report contains the collective views of an international group of experts and does not necessarily represent the decisions or the stated policy of the United Nations Environment Programme, the International Labour Organisation, or the World Health Organization

**Environmental Health Criteria 97**

# DELTAMETHRIN

Published under the joint sponsorship of the United Nations Environment Programme, the International Labour Organisation, and the World Health Organization

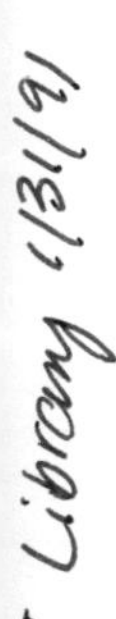


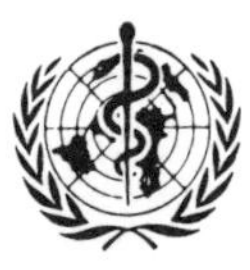

World Health Organization
Geneva, 1990

The International Programme on Chemical Safety (IPCS) is a joint venture of the United Nations Environment Programme, the International Labour Organisation, and the World Health Organization. The main objective of the IPCS is to carry out and disseminate evaluations of the effects of chemicals on human health and the quality of the environment. Supporting activities include the development of epidemiological, experimental laboratory, and risk-assessment methods that could produce internationally comparable results, and the development of manpower in the field of toxicology. Other activities carried out by the IPCS include the development of know-how for coping with chemical accidents, coordination of laboratory testing and epidemiological studies, and promotion of research on the mechanisms of the biological action of chemicals.

WHO Library Cataloguing in Publication Data

Deltamethrin

(Environmental health criteria ; 97)

1.Pyrethrins I.Series

ISBN 92 4 154297 7 (NLM Classification: WA 240)
ISSN 0250-863X



The designations employed and the presentation of the material in this publication do not imply the expression of any opinion whatsoever on the part of the Secretariat of the World Health Organization concerning the legal status of any country, territory, city or area or of its authorities, or concerning the delimitation of its frontiers or boundaries.

The mention of specific companies or of certain manufacturers' products does not imply that they are endorsed or recommended by the World Health Organization in preference to others of a similar nature that are not mentioned. Errors and omissions excepted, the names of proprietary products are distinguished by initial capital letters.

Computer typesetting by HEADS, Oxford OX7 2NY, England

PRINTED IN FINLAND
Vammalan Kirjapaino Oy
DHSS — Vammala — 5000

# CONTENTS

# WHO TASK GROUP ON ENVIRONMENTAL HEALTH CRITERIA FOR TETRAMETHRIN, CYHALOTHRIN, AND DELTAMETHRIN

*Members*

Dr V. Benes, Department of Toxicology & Reference Laboratory, Institute of Hygiene and Epidemiology, Prague, Czechoslovakia

Dr A.J. Browning, Toxicology Evaluation Section, Department of Community Services and Health, Woden, Australia

Dr S. Dobson, Institute of Terrestrial Ecology, Monks Wood Experimental Station, Huntingdon, Cambridge, United Kingdom (*Chairman*)

Dr K. Imaida, Section of Tumor Pathology, Division of Pathology, National Institute of Hygienic Sciences, Tokyo, Japan

Dr P. Hurley, Office of Pesticide Programme, US Environmental Protection Agency, Washington, DC, USA

Dr S.K. Kashyap, National Institute of Occupational Health, (I.C.M.R.) Ahmedabad, India (*Vice-Chairman*)

Dr Yu. I. Kundiev, Research Institute of Labour, Hygiene and Occupational Diseases, Kiev, USSR

Dr J.P. Leahey, ICI Agrochemicals, Jealotts Hill Research Station, Bracknell, Berkshire, United Kingdom (*Rapporteur*)

Dr M. Matsuo, Sumitomo Chemical Company Limited, Biochemistry & Toxicology Laboratory, Osaka, Japan

*Observers*

Mr M. L'Hotellier, International Group of National Associations of Manufacturers of Agrochemical Products (GIFAP)

Dr N. Punja, International Group of National Associations of Manufacturers of Agrochemical Products (GIFAP)

*Secretariat*

Dr K.W. Jager, Division of Environmental Health, International Programme on Chemical Safety, World Health Organization, Geneva, Switzerland (*Secretary*)

Dr R. Plestina, Division of Vector Biology and Control, World Health Organization, Geneva, Switzerland

Dr J. Sekizawa, Division of Information on Chemical Safety, National Institute of Hygienic Sciences, Tokyo, Japan (*Rapporteur*)

# NOTE TO READERS OF THE CRITERIA DOCUMENTS

Every effort has been made to present information in the criteria documents as accurately as possible without unduly delaying their publication. In the interest of all users of the environmental health criteria documents, readers are kindly requested to communicate any errors that may have occurred to the Manager of the International Programme on Chemical Safety, World Health Organization, Geneva, Switzerland, in order that they may be included in corrigenda, which will appear in subsequent volumes.

* * *

A detailed data profile and a legal file can be obtained from the International Register of Potentially Toxic Chemicals, Palais des Nations, 1211 Geneva 10, Switzerland (Telephone no. 7988400 - 7985850).

NOTE

The proprietary information contained in this document cannot replace documentation for registration purposes, because the latter has to be closely linked to the source, the manufacturing route, and the purity/impurities of the substance to be registered. The data should be used in accordance with para. 82-84 and recommendations para 90 of the 2nd FAO Government Consultation (1982).

# ENVIRONMENTAL HEALTH CRITERIA FOR TETRAMETHRIN, CYHALOTHRIN, AND DELTAMETHRIN

A WHO Task Group on Environmental Health Criteria for Tetramethrin, Cyhalothrin, and Deltamethrin met at the World Health Organization, Geneva, from 24–28 October 1988. Dr M. Mercier, Manager of the IPCS, welcomed the participants on behalf of the three IPCS cooperating organizations (UNEP/ILO/WHO). The Group reviewed and revised the draft Criteria Documents and Health and Safety Guides and made an evaluation of the risks for human health and the environment from exposure to tetramethrin, cyhalothrin, and deltamethrin.

The first drafts of the documents on tetramethrin and deltamethrin were prepared by Dr J. MIYAMOTO and Dr M. MATSUO of Sumitomo Chemical Co. Limited. Dr J. SEKIZAWA of the National Institute of Hygienic Sciences, Tokyo, Japan, assisted in the finalization of the drafts. The first draft of the document on cyhalothrin was prepared by the IPCS Secretariat based on material made available by ICI Agrochemicals, United Kingdom.

The second drafts were prepared by the IPCS Secretariat, incorporating comments received following circulation of the first drafts to the IPCS contact points for Environmental Health Criteria documents.

Dr K.W. JAGER of the IPCS Central Unit was responsible for the scientific content of the deltamethrin document, and Mrs M.O. HEAD of Oxford, England, for the editing.

The fact that Sumitomo Chemical Company Limited, Japan, ICI Agrochemicals, United Kingdom, and Roussel Uclaf SA, France, made available to the IPCS and the Task Group their proprietary toxicological information on their products under discussion is gratefully acknowledged. This allowed the Task Group to make their evaluation on a more complete data base.

The effort of all who helped in the preparation and finalization of the documents is gratefully acknowledged.

# INTRODUCTION

## Synthetic pyrethroids – a profile

During investigations to modify the chemical structures of natural pyrethrins, a certain number of synthetic pyrethroids were produced with improved physical and chemical properties and greater biological activity. Several of the earlier synthetic pyrethroids were successfully commercialized, mainly for the control of household insects. Other more recent pyrethroids have been introduced as agricultural insecticides because of their excellent activity against a wide range of insect pests and their non-persistence in the environment.

The pyrethroids constitute another group of insecticides in addition to organochlorine, organophosphorus, carbamate, and other compounds. Pyrethroids commercially available so far include allethrin, resmethrin, d-phenothrin, and tetramethrin (for insects of public health importance), and cypermethrin, deltamethrin, fenvalerate, and permethrin (mainly for agricultural insects). Other pyrethroids are also available, including furamethrin, kadethrin, and tellallethrin (usually for household insects), fenpropathrin, tralomethrin, cyhalothrin, lambda-cyhalothrin, tefluthrin, cyfluthrin, flucythrinate, fluvalinate, and biphenate (for agricultural insects).

Toxicological evaluations of several synthetic pyrethroids have been performed by the FAO/WHO Joint Meeting on Pesticide Residues (JMPR). The acceptable daily intake (ADI) has been estimated by the JMPR for cypermethrin, deltamethrin, fenvalerate, permethrin, d-phenothrin, cyfluthrin, cyhalothrin, and flucythrinate.

Chemically, synthetic pyrethroids are esters of specific acids (e.g., chrysanthemic acid, halo-substituted chrysanthemic acid, 2-(4-chlorophenyl)-3-methylbutyric acid) and alcohols (e.g., allethrolone, 3-phenoxybenzyl alcohol). For certain pyrethroids, the asymmetric centre(s) exist in the acid and/or alcohol moiety, and the commercial products sometimes consist of a mixture of both optical (1R/1S or *d*/*l*) and geometric (*cis*/*trans*) isomers. However, most of the insecticidal activity of such products may reside in only one or two isomers. Some of the products (e.g., d-phenothrin, deltamethrin) consist only of such active isomer(s).

Synthetic pyrethroids are neuropoisons acting on the axons in the peripheral and central nervous systems by interacting with sodium channels in mammals and/or insects. A single dose produces toxic signs in mammals, such as tremors, hyper-excitability, salivation, choreo-athetosis, and paralysis. The signs disappear fairly rapidly, and the animals recover, generally within a week. At near-lethal dose levels, synthetic pyrethroids cause transient changes in the nervous system, such as axonal swelling and/or breaks and myelin degeneration in the sciatic nerves. They are not considered to cause delayed neurotoxicity of the kind induced by some organophosphorus compounds. The mechanism of toxicity of synthetic pyrethroids, and their classification into two types, are discussed in Appendix 1.

Some pyrethroids (e.g., deltamethrin, fenvalerate, flucythrinate, and cypermethrin) may cause a transient itching and/or burning sensation in exposed human skin.

Synthetic pyrethroids are generally metabolized in mammals through ester hydrolysis, oxidation, and conjugation, and there is no tendency to accumulate in tissues. In the environment, synthetic pyrethroids are fairly rapidly degraded in soil and in plants. Ester hydrolysis and oxidation at various sites on the molecule are the major degradation processes. The pyrethroids are strongly adsorbed on soil and sediments, and are hardly eluted with water. There is little tendency for bioaccumulation in organisms.

Because of low application rates and rapid degradation in the environment, residues in food are generally low.

Synthetic pyrethroids have been shown to be toxic for fish, aquatic arthropods, and honey-bees in laboratory tests. But, in practical usage, no serious adverse effects have been noticed because of the low rates of application and lack of persistence in the environment. The toxicity of synthetic pyrethroids in birds and domestic animals is low.

In addition to the evaluation documents of FAO/WHO, there are several good reviews and books on the chemistry, metabolism, mammalian toxicity, environmental effects, etc., of synthetic pyrethroids, including those by Elliot (1977), Miyamoto (1981), Miyamoto & Kearney (1983), and Leahey (1985).

# 1. SUMMARY AND EVALUATION, CONCLUSIONS AND RECOMMENDATIONS

## 1.1 Summary and evaluation

### *1.1.1 Identity, physical and chemical properties, analytical methods*

Deltamethrin was synthesized in 1974, and first marketed in 1977. Chemically, it is the [1R,*cis*; αS]-isomer of 8 stereoisomeric esters of the dibromo analogue of chrysanthemic acid, 2,2-dimethyl-3-(2,2-dibromovinyl) cyclopropanecarboxylic acid ($Br_2CA$) with α-cyano-3 phenoxybenzyl alcohol.

Technical grade deltamethrin is an odourless white powder with a melting point of 98–101 °C and contains more than 98% of the material. The vapour pressure is $2.0 \times 10^{-6}$ Pa at 25 °C and it is practically non-volatile. It is insoluble in water, but soluble in organic solvents, such as acetone, cyclohexanone, and xylene. It is stable to light, heat, and air, but unstable in alkaline media.

The determination of residues and analysis of environmental samples were carried out by solvent extraction with *n*-hexane/acetone, partitioning with *n*-hexane/acetone/water, clean-up with a silica gel column chromatograph, and determination with a gas chromatograph equipped with an electron capture detector with a minimum detectable concentration of 0.01 mg/kg or less. High-performance liquid chromatography with an UV-detector is used for product analysis.

### *1.1.2 Production and uses*

The consumption of deltamethrin in the world was about 250 tonnes in 1987. It is mostly used on cotton (45 % of the consumption) and on crops such as coffee, maize, cereals, fruit, vegetables, and hops, and on stored products. Deltamethrin is also used in animal health, in vector control, and in public health. It is formulated as an emulsifiable concentrate, ultra-low-volume concentrate, wettable powder, suspension concentrate, or dust powder, alone, or in combination with other pesticides.

### 1.1.3 Human exposure

Exposure of the general population to deltamethrin is mainly via dietary residues, but may also occur from its use in public health. Residue levels in crops treated according to good agricultural practice are generally very low, except for those arising from post-harvest treatment. Extensive data have been reviewed by FAO/WHO (see page 89).

Exposure of the general population is expected to be very low, but actual data in the form of total diet studies are lacking.

### 1.1.4 Environmental exposure and fate

When $^{14}$C-(acid, alcohol, or cyano labelling)-deltamethrin-[1R, *cis*; αS] was exposed to sunlight as a thin film for 4–8 h, 70% of it was transformed by *cis/trans*-isomerization to give the [1R, *trans*; αS] and [1S, *trans;* αS] isomers, together with ester cleavage products, including $Br_2CA$ and α-cyano-3-phenoxybenzyl alcohol.

Deltamethrin was degraded in cotton plants, under glasshouse conditions, with an initial half-life of 1.1 weeks, and the time needed for 90% loss was 4.6 weeks.

The major metabolites were free and conjugated $Br_2CA$, *trans*-hydroxymethyl-$Br_2CA$, and 3-(4-hydroxyphenoxy)benzoic acid formed by ester cleavage, oxidation, and conjugation.

Deltamethrin was incubated in sand and organic soil at 28 °C under laboratory conditions. Approximately 52% and 74% of the applied deltamethrin was recovered from sand and organic soil, respectively, 8 weeks after treatment.

Deltamethrin is not mobile in the environment because of its strong adsorption on particles, its insolubility in water, and very low rates of application.

No data are available on actual levels in the environment, but with the current use pattern and under normal conditions of use, environmental exposure is expected to be very low. Degradation to less toxic products is rapid.

### 1.1.5 Uptake, metabolism, and excretion

Deltamethrin is readily absorbed by the oral route, but less so dermally; the rate of absorption is strongly dependent on the carrier or solvent. Absorbed deltamethrin is readily metabolized and excreted.

When rats were given $^{14}C$-(acid, alcohol, or cyano labelled)-deltamethrin orally at the rate of 0.64–1.60 mg/kg, the radiocarbon from the acid and alcohol moiety was almost completely eliminated within 2–4 days. Tissue residue levels were generally very low, except in fat, where slightly higher residues occurred. However, the cyano portion was excreted more slowly, with total recovery of 79% in 8 days. The major metabolic reactions were oxidation (at the *trans*-methyl of the cyclopropane ring and at the 2′-, 4′-, and 5-positions of the alcohol moiety), ester cleavage, and conversion of the cyano portion to thiocyanate. The resultant carboxylic acids and phenols were conjugated with sulfuric acid, glycine, and glucuronic acid.

When mice were fed $^{14}C$-(acid, alcohol, or cyano labelled)-deltamethrin orally at rates of 1.7–4.4 mg/kg, the excretion of the radiocarbon was rapid and almost complete, except for the cyano portion. The major metabolic reactions in mice were generally similar to those in rats.

In cows and poultry, degradation pathways are very close to those in rodents.

### 1.1.6 Effects on organisms in the environment

Deltamethrin is highly toxic for fish, the 96-h $LC_{50}$ ranging between 0.4 and 2.0 µg/litre. It is also highly toxic for aquatic invertebrates; the 48-h $LC_{50}$ for *Daphnia* is 5 µg/litre. However, extensive field studies, in experimental ponds, and field use have shown that this high potential toxicity is not realized. Some kills of aquatic invertebrates occur in the field, but these are usually compensated for rapidly.

The toxicity of deltamethrin for birds is very low with $LD_{50}$ values for a single oral dose exceeding 1000 mg/kg. Under laboratory conditions, it is highly toxic for honey-bees with a contact $LD_{50}$ of 0.051 µg/bee. Field trials and actual usage have established that deltamethrin formulations have a repellent action, which means that, in practice, the hazard for bees is low.

### 1.1.7 *Effects on experimental animals and* in vitro *test systems*

In a non-aqueous vehicle, the acute oral toxicity of deltamethrin is high to moderate with $LD_{50}$ values of 19–34 mg/kg (mouse) and 31–139 mg/kg (rat). However, in a suspension in water, the toxicity is much less with $LD_{50}$ values exceeding 5000 mg/kg (rat). Deltamethrin is a Type II pyrethroid; clinical signs of poisoning include tremor, salivation, and convulsion. The onset of signs is rapid and they disappear within several days in survivors. The electroencephalogram shows generalized spike and wave discharges prior to choreo-athetosis.

Single applications of technical deltamethrin did not produce any irritant effect on the intact and abraded skin of the rabbit. However, transient irritating effects were produced in the eye of the rabbit, with and without rinsing. Deltamethrin was not a skin sensitizer in the guinea-pig.

When rats were dosed, by gavage, with deltamethrin levels of up to 10.0 mg/kg body weight per day for 13 weeks, hyperexcitability was observed at 6 weeks in males given the highest dose. Body weight gain was lower in males given 2.5 and 10 mg/kg.

When beagle dogs were dosed orally with deltamethrin at levels of up to 10 mg/kg body weight per day for 13 weeks, there were various compound-related symptoms, such as vomiting, tremor, salivation, and depressed gag- , patellar- , and flexor reflexes. In a 2-year feeding study on dogs, 1 mg/kg body weight per day was the no-observed-effect level (highest level tested).

When mice were fed deltamethrin at levels of up to 100 mg/kg diet for 24 months, tumour incidence was unaffected. The no-observed-effect level for systemic toxicity was 100 mg/kg diet.

When rats were fed deltamethrin at levels of up to 50 mg/kg diet for 2 years, no compound-related tumours were observed. The no-observed-effect level for systemic toxicity was 50 mg/kg diet.

Deltamethrin was not mutagenic in a variety of *in vivo* and *in vitro* test systems, including: DNA repair, gene mutation, chromosomal aberration, sister chromatid exchange, micronucleus formation, and dominant lethal tests.

Teratology studies were conducted on pregnant rats and mice in which deltamethrin was administered orally at levels of up to 10 mg/kg body weight per day during the period of major organogenesis. There were no teratogenic or reproductive effects, except for a dose-related decrease in mean fetal weight in the mouse study and slightly delayed ossification in the rat study.

Rabbits received deltamethrin at levels of up to 16 mg/kg body weight per day between days 6 and 19 of pregnancy. A decreased average fetal weight was noted at the highest dose. No teratogenic effects were observed in rabbits.

When rats were fed deltamethrin at levels of up to 50 mg/kg diet in a 3-generation, 2-litter reproduction study, no effects on reproduction were observed.

There are indications that potentiation of toxicity may occur when deltamethrin is combined with some organophosphorus compounds.

### 1.1.8 Effects on human beings

Deltamethrin can induce skin sensations in exposed workers. Several non-fatal cases of poisoning have been reported through occupational exposure resulting from neglect of safety precautions. Numbness, itching, tingling, and burning of the skin and vertigo are symptoms that are frequently reported. Occasionally, a transient papular or blotchy erythema has been described. Most of these symptoms are transient and disappear within 5–7 days. No long-term adverse effects have been reported. Three non-fatal cases of deltamethrin poisoning have been described following ingestion of several grams of the product.

## 1.2 Conclusions

*General population*: The exposure of the general population to deltamethrin is expected to be very low and is not likely to present a hazard under recommended conditions of use.

*Occupational exposure*: With good work practices, measures of hygiene, and safety precautions, deltamethrin is unlikely to present a hazard for those occupationally exposed.

*Environment*: It is unlikely that deltamethrin or its degradation products will attain levels of adverse environmental significance with recommended rates of application. Under laboratory conditions, deltamethrin is highly toxic for fish, aquatic arthropods, and honey-bees. However, under field conditions, lasting adverse effects are not likely to occur under recommended conditions of use.

## 1.3 Recommendations

Although dietary levels are considered to be very low following recommended usage, confirmation of this through inclusion of deltamethrin in monitoring studies should be considered.

Deltamethrin has been used for many years and several cases of non-fatal poisoning and transient effects from occupational exposure have been reported. Observations of human exposure should be maintained.

# 2. IDENTITY, PHYSICAL AND CHEMICAL PROPERTIES, ANALYTICAL METHODS

## 2.1 Identity

Molecular formula: $C_{22}H_{19}Br_2NO_3$

Chemical formula:

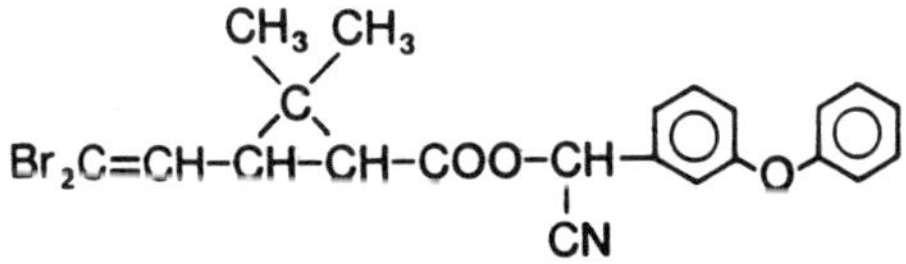

$Br_2C{=}CH{-}CH{-}CH{-}COO{-}CH(CN){-}C_6H_4{-}O{-}C_6H_5$ (cyclopropane ring bearing C($CH_3$)($CH_3$))

Chemical structure of 8 stereoisomers:

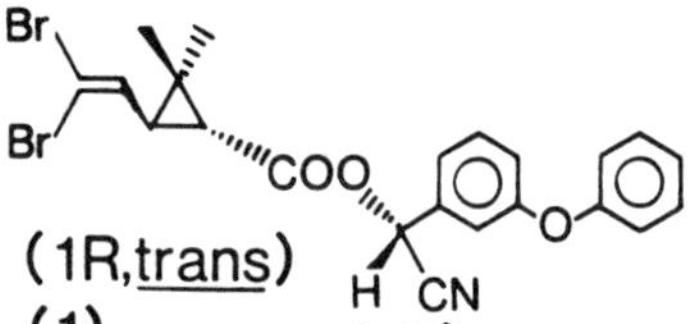

(1R,trans) (αR) (1)

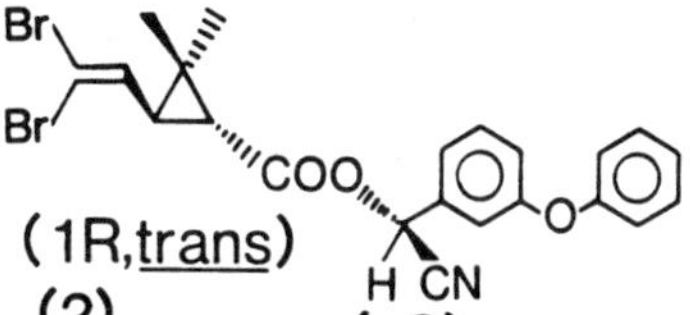

(1R,trans) (αS) (2)

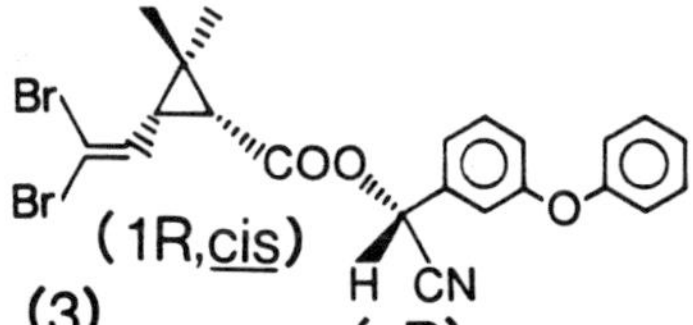

(1R,cis) (αR) (3)

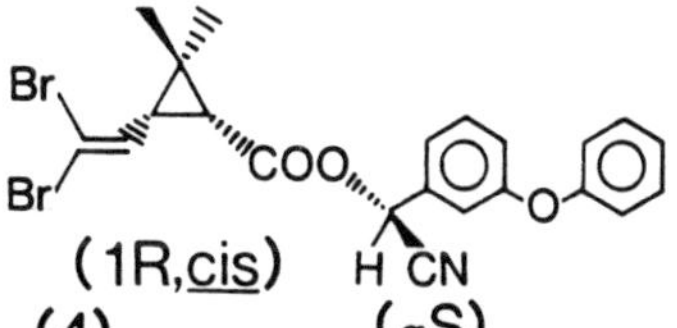

(1R,cis) (αS) (4)

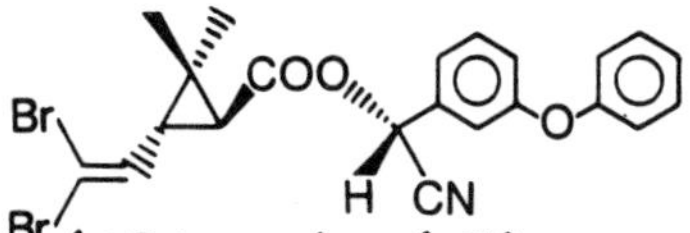

(1S,trans) (αR) (5)

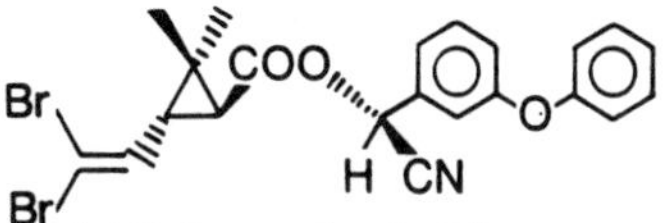

(1S,trans) (αS) (6)

Chemical structure of 8 stereoisomers (*continued*):

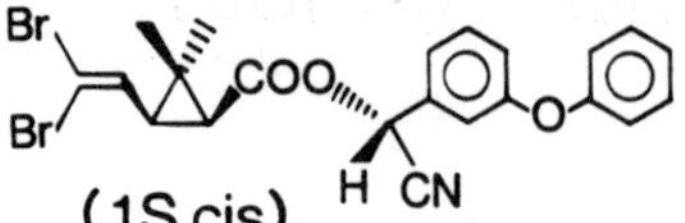

Br Br COO O H CN (1S,cis) (αR) (7)

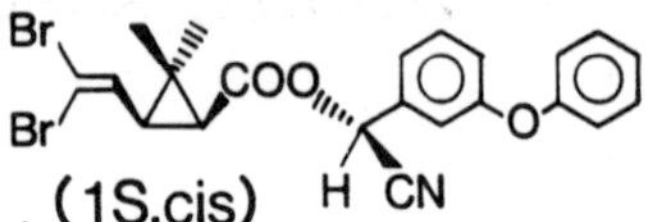

Br Br COO O H CN (1S,cis) (αS) (8)

Deltamethrin is the first pyrethroid composed of a single isomer of 8 stereoisomers selectively prepared by the esterification of [1R, 3R or *cis*]-2,2-dimethyl-3-(2,2-dibromovinyl) cyclopropane-carboxylic acid with (αS)- or (+)-α-cyano-3-phenoxybenzyl alcohol or by selective recrystallization of the racemic esters obtained by esterification of the (1R, 3R or *cis*)-acid with the racemic or [αR, αS, or αRS or ±]-alcohol (Elliott et al., 1974). Thus, its stereospecific structure (4) is the ester of [1R, 3R or *cis*]-acid with (αS)-alcohol.

The acid is a characteristic dibromo analogue of chrysanthemic acid.

## 2.2 Physical and chemical properties

Technical grade deltamethrin contains more than 98% deltamethrin (FAO/WHO, 1981). It is stable to heat (6 months at 40 °C), light, and air, but unstable in alkaline media (FAO/WHO, 1981; Meister et al., 1983; Worthing & Walker, 1983). Some physical and chemical properties are listed in Table 1, and the chemical composition of various stereoisomeric mixtures is shown in Table 2.

## 2.3 Analytical methods

Methods for the determination of deltamethrin residues and the analysis of environmental samples and products are summarized in Table 3.

To analyse technical grade deltamethrin, a mixture of deltamethrin and diphenylamine (an internal standard) was injected in a high-performance liquid chromatograph equipped with a UV-detector (Mourot et al., 1979).

Table 1. Some physical and chemical properties of deltamethrin

| | |
|---|---|
| Physical state | crystalline powder |
| Colour | colourless |
| Odour | odourless |
| Density (20 °C) | 0.5 g/cm$^3$ |
| Relative molecular mass | 505.24 |
| Melting point (°C) | 98–101 |
| Boiling point | decomposes above 300 °C |
| Water solubility (20 °C) | < 0.002 mg/litre (practically insoluble) |
| Solubility in organic solvents | soluble[a] |
| Vapour pressure (25 °C) | 2.0 x $10^{-6}$ Pa |
| *n*-Octanol-water partition coefficient (Log Pow) | 5.43 |

[a] Acetone (500 g/litre), ethanol (15 g/litre), cyclohexanone (750 g/litre), dioxane (900 g/litre), xylene (250 g/litre), ethyl acetate.

The Joint FAO/WHO Codex Alimentarius Commission has published recommendations for methods for the determination of deltamethrin residues (FAO/WHO 1985b). A further review of analytical methods for deltamethrin has been made by Vaysse et al. (1984).

Table 2. Chemical identity of deltamethrins of various stereoisomeric compositions

| Common name<br>CAS Registry No.<br>NIOSH Accession No.[a] | CA Index name (9CI)<br><br>Stereospecific name[b] | Stereoisomeric composition[c] | Synonyms and trade names |
|---|---|---|---|
| Deltamethrin<br>52918-63-5<br>GZ1233000*a* | Cyclopropanecarboxylic acid,<br>3-(2,2-dibromovinyl)-2,2-dimethyl-,<br>α-cyano(3-phenoxyphenyl)methyl ester,<br>[1R-[1 (S*), 3 R]]-,<br><br>(S)-α-cyano-3-phenoxybenzyl<br>(1R, *cis*)-2,2-dimethyl-3-(2,2-di-<br>bromovinyl)cyclopropanecarboxylate | (4) | Decamethrin, Decis,<br>K-Othrine, NRDC 161,<br>WHO 1998, K-Obiol, Butox<br>Butoflin, Cislin, FMC 45498<br>RU 22974 |
| d-*cis*-Deltamethrin<br>52820-00-5<br>GZ1240000*a* | same as deltamethrin<br><br>(S)-α-cyano-3-phenoxybenzyl<br>(d, *cis*)-2,2-dimethyl-3-(2,2-di-<br>bromovinyl)cyclopropanecarboxylate | - | Decamethrin, Decis |

[a] Registry of Toxic Effects of Chemical Substances (RTECS) (1981–82 edition).
[b] (1R), d, (+) or (1S), 1, (-) in the acid part of deltamethrin signifies the same stereospecific conformation, respectively.
[c] The number in the parenthesis identifies the structure shown in the figures of stereoisomers.

Table 3. Analytical methods for deltamethrin

| Sample | Extraction solvent | Sample preparation | | | Determination: | MDC[b] (mg/kg) | % Recovery (fortification level in mg/kg) | Reference |
|---|---|---|---|---|---|---|---|---|
| | | Partition | Clean up | | GLC or HPLC condition; detector, carrier flow, column, temp, R.T.[a] | | | |
| | | | column | elution | | | | |
| RESIDUE ANALYSIS | | | | | | | | |
| apple | *n*-hexane/ acetone (1/1) | ext.sol.[c] /$H_2O$ | silica gel | $CH_2Cl_2$ | ECD–GC; $N_2$; 50 ml/min; 1 m 3% OV-7; 235 °C | 0.01 | 105(0.1), 100(1.0) | 1 |
| pear | | | | | | 0.01 | 125(0.1), 98(1.0) | |
| cabbage | | | | | | 0.01 | 130(0.1), 118(1.0) | |
| potato | | | | | | 0.01 | 126(0.1), 97(1.0) | |
| apple, peach, grape, tomato | acetonitrile | petro- leum ether/ $H_2O$ | Florisil | ether/ *n*-hexane (1/4) | EDC-GC; 1.2 m DC-200, OV-1 or OV-101; 245 °C, 10–12 min | 0.005 | 85–100(0.02–0.1) | 2 |
| wheat grain | methanol | *n*-hexane | alumina | | HPLC; 235 nm; 30 cm; uBondapak; C 18; methanol/$H_2O$ (4/1); 2.5 ml/min | | 87(2.0) | 3 |
| wheat | *n*-hexane | | Florisil | ether/ petro- leum ether (1/9) | ECD–GC; $N_2$; 75 ml/min; 0.6 m 5% SE-30; 215 °C | | 91 | 4 |

Table 3 (*continued*)

| Sample | Extraction solvent | Sample preparation | | | Dermination: GLC or HPLC condition; detector, carrier flow, column, temp, R..T.[a] | MDC[b] (mg/kg) | % Recovery (fortification level in mg/kg) | Reference |
|---|---|---|---|---|---|---|---|---|
| | | Partition | Clean up: column | Clean up: elution | | | | |
| meat | ethyl ether/ petroleum ether | acetonitrile | gel permeation column (Styragel) | diisopropyl ether | ECD–GLC; $N_2$; 40ml/min; 1.8 m SE-30 1% on gas Chrom. PAW | 0.001 | 90–95% at 0.01 | 5 |
| milk | hexane | acetonitrile | Florisil + cellulose/ charcoal | benzene/ hexane (1/1) | ECD–GLC; $N_2$; 40 ml/min; 1.8 m SE-30 1% on gas Chrom. PAW | 0.01 | 83–87% at 0.1 | 5 |
| ENVIRONMENTAL ANALYSIS | | | | | | | | |
| locust | *n*-hexane | | Florisil | ether/ petroleum ether (1/9) | ECD–GC; $N_2$; 75 ml/min; 0.6 m 5% SE-30; 215 °C | | 92 | 4 |
| sea water | XAD-2 resin acetone | ext.sol.[c]/ *n*-hexane | alumina | | ECD–GC; $N_2$; 70 ml/min; 1.5 m 4% SE-30; 207 °C | | | 6 |

Table 3 (*continued*)

| | | | | | | | |
|---|---|---|---|---|---|---|---|
| water | *n*-hexane | alumina | | ECD–GC; $N_2$; 70 ml/min; 1.5 m 4% SE-30; 207 °C | | | 6 |
| water | petroleum ether/ diethyl-ether (1/1) | Florisil | petroleum ether/ diethyl-ether (80/20) | ECD–GLC; 1m OV 1-3% on Chromo-sorb W.A.W. HMDS 60/80 | 0.0001 | 97 at 0.010 | 8 |
| soil | acetone, acetone/ hexane (1/1) hexane | acid alumina | hexane ether hexane (5-10%) | ECD–GLC: 5.2% OV-210 with AR/CH4 | 0.001 | > 91% | 9 |
| | acetone, acetone/ hexane (1/1) hexane | acid alumina | hexane/ ethyl-ether (90/10) | ECD–GLC; $N_2$; 40 ml/min; 1.8 m SE-30 1% on gas Chrom. PAW | 0.0001 | > 91% | 5 |
| cotton foliage (dislodgeable residue) | *n*-hexane | | | transesterification followed by ECD–GC; 31 ml/min; 0.45 m 5% SE-30; 120 °C | | | 7 |

Table 3 (*continued*)

| Sample | Extraction solvent | Sample preparation | | | Dermination: GLC or HPLC condition; detector, carrier flow, column, temp, R..T.[a] | MDC[b] (mg/kg) | % Recovery (fortification level in mg/kg) | Reference |
|---|---|---|---|---|---|---|---|---|
| | | Partition | Clean up | | | | | |
| | | | column | elution | | | | |
| PRODUCT ANALYSIS | | | | | | | | |
| Technical grade | | | | | HPLC, 230 nm; 15 cm Lichrosorb Si-60; *n*-hexane/ diisopropyl ether (93/7); 80 ml/h; 7.6 min | | | 10 |
| | isoctane/ dioxane (80/20) | | | | HPLC - UV detector 254 nm (230 nm for conc. <0.5%) Silica-60; 100ml/h; isooctane/ dioxane (95/5) | | | 5 |

[a] R.T. : retention time; [b] MDC : minimum detectable concentration; [c] ext .sol. : extraction solvent.

References

1. Baker & Bottomley (1982); 2. Mestres et al. (1978a); 3. Noble et al. (1982); 4. Pansu et al. (1981); 5. Vaysse et al. (1984); 6. Zitko et al. (1979); 7. Estesen et al. (1979); 8. Mestres et al. (1978b); 9. Hill (1982); 10. Mourot et al. (1979).

# 3. SOURCES OF ENVIRONMENTAL POLLUTION AND ENVIRONMENTAL LEVELS

## 3.1 Industrial production

Deltamethrin was first marketed in 1977. Production volumes in recent years are shown in Table 4.

Table 4. Worldwide production of deltamethrin

| Year | Production (tonnes) | Reference |
| --- | --- | --- |
| 1979 | 75 | Wood Mackenzie (1980) |
| 1980 | 100 | Wood Mackenzie (1981) |
| 1981 | 100 | Wood Mackenzie (1982, 1983) |
| 1982 | 115 | Wood Mackenzie (1983) |
| 1987 | 250 | Information from Roussel Uclaf |

## 3.2 Use patterns

After an initial period when the product was mainly used on cotton, several major crops were treated with deltamethrin from 1980 to 1987. Some 85% of the total production is used for crop protection. Within this, 45 % is used on cotton, 25% on fruit and vegetable crops, 20% on cereals, corn, and soybean, and the remaining 10% on miscellaneous crops.

Deltamethrin is used to protect stored commodities (mainly cereals, grains, coffee beans, dry beans), in forestry, and in public health (e.g., Chagas disease control in South America, and malaria control in Central America and on the African continent). It is also used in animal facilities and against cattle infestation.

It is formulated as an emulsifable concentrate (25–100 g/litre), an ultra-low-volume concentrate (1.5–30 g/litre), a wettable powder (25–50 g/kg), a flowable powder (7.5–50 g/litre), or a dust powder (0.5–2.5 g/kg). It is also used in combination with other pesticides and with piperonyl butoxide (unpublished information from Roussel Uclaf to the IPCS, 1988).

## 3.3 Residues in food

Supervised trials have been carried out on a wide variety of crops and comprehensive summaries of analyses for residues in these trials can be found in the evaluation reports of the Joint FAO/WHO Meeting on Pesticide Residues (JMPR) (FAO/WHO 1981, 1982, 1983, 1985a, 1986a, 1986b, 1988b). A comprehensive list of maximum residue limits (MRLs) for a large number of commodities resulted from these evaluations (FAO/WHO, 1986c, 1988a,c) (see section 9).

Residues were determined in stored products, e.g., wheat, maize, and coffee. The residue level in wheat grains treated with deltamethrin at the rate of 2 mg/kg was 1.08 mg/kg after storage for 9 months. When the wheat was subjected to milling and baking, the residue levels in white bread were 0.11 mg/kg (Halls & Periam, 1980).

Mestres et al. (1986) reviewed the changes in deltamethrin residues in edible crops resulting from processing and cooking and found that, depending on the commodity, pre- or post-harvest residues were reduced by 20–98% by processing, and especially by cooking.

When 0.27 g of $^{14}$C-(alcohol labelling)-deltamethrin was injected intrarumenally in a lactating Jersey cow, in solution in a sesame oil/alcohol mixture, only 0.4% of the compound was found in whole milk. Peak residue levels of 0.045 and 0.92 mg/kg were found in whole milk and rendered butter fat, respectively, 1 day after administration. Residues in omental fat and leg muscle were 0.088 and 0.008 mg/kg, respectively, 2 days after treatment (Wellcome Foundation, 1979).

## 3.4 Levels in the environment

No information is available.

# 4. ENVIRONMENTAL TRANSPORT, DISTRIBUTION, AND TRANSFORMATION

## 4.1 Transport and distribution between media

Using three different soils (silty clay, silty clay loam, and loamy sand), Kaufman et al. (1981) found that deltamethrin was practically immobile in soil columns. Approximately 96–97% of the $^{14}C$ activity remained in the upper 0–2.5 cm layer of the columns with only 1.3 % in the 2.5–5.1 cm layer and no $^{14}C$ in the leachate. Soil thin layer chromatography (soil TLC) was also used to evaluate the mobility of deltamethrin. According to the pesticide mobility classification system developed by Helling & Turner, deltamethrin is classified as a low-mobility to immobile compound in soils.

The immobility of deltamethrin in soil was also studied by Hascoet (1977) using a French Fontainebleau sand column leached with a very high volume of water (equivalent to 1030 mm of rain). In this experiment, approximately 97% of the applied $^{14}C$-deltamethrin remained in the upper 0–2.5 cm layer and only 2% was found in the leachate. The author concluded that deltamethrin was unlikely to leach in cultivated soil that had a higher organic matter content and/or higher clay contents than sand (organic matter 0.03%), which has especially good filtration and low adsorption properties.

The leaching of deltamethrin was also studied in three different German soils the organic contents of which ranged from 0.8 to 2.6%. The study was carried out using the commercial product Decis EC 25 at a rate equivalent to 1 litre/ha (i.e., 25 g deltamethrin/ha). Each column was leached with 370 ml of water, which was equivalent to a rainfall of 200 mm for 2 days. Under these conditions, the amount of active ingredient (a.i.) detected in seepage water was found to be less than 1 μg/ml, which was less than 2% of the original applied dose (Thier & Schmidt, 1976).

The mobility of the primary deltamethrin degradation products 3-phenoxybenzoic acid (PBacid) and 3-phenoxybenzyl alcohol (PBalc) was also investigated by Kaufman et al. (1981) using soil TLC and soil columns. PBacid was found to be relatively mobile, whereas PBalc was only slightly mobile. 2,2-Dimethyl-3-(2,2-dibromovinyl) cyclopropanecarboxylic acid ($Br_2CA$) was not studied in this experiment, but $Cl_2CA$, the chloride substituted analogue, was evaluated and also found to be relatively mobile. However, these metabolites did not accumulate in the soil to any extent, since they were never in excess of 3% of the applied dose under the aerobic conditions reported by Kaufman & Kayser (1979a,b). The very significant production of $^{14}CO_2$ during the incubation period confirmed that they were further degraded.

## 4.2 Abiotic degradation in air and water

Degradation pathways for deltamethrin are summarized in Fig.1.

When $^{14}$C-deltamethrin-[1R, 3R; αS] (9) labelled at the cyano, benzylic, or dibromo-substituted carbon was exposed to sunlight as a thin film (40 μg/cm$^2$) for 4-8 h, the *trans*-[1R, 3S; αS] and -[1S, 3R; αS] isomers were formed. They accounted for approximately 70% of the applied radioactivity. Smaller amounts of ester cleavage products including the 2,2-dimethyl-3-(2,2-dibromovinyl) cyclopropanecarboxylic acid ($Br_2CA$) (18) and the cyanohydrin component, and 18% of unidentified products were also formed (Fig. 1). In a thick film (3 mg/cm$^2$), small amounts of other products including α-cyano-3-phenoxybenzyl 3,3-dimethylacrylate (13) and 3-phenoxy 2,2-dimethyl-3-(2,2-dibromovinyl)cyclopropan-1-yl-benzylcyanide (14) (decarboxy-deltamethrin) were also detected. In contrast, the predominant products in methanol were the *trans* mixtures, which amounted to approximately 35% of the applied radioactivity. Under UV radiation (peak output 290–320 nm), the photodegradation rate of deltamethrin in alcohols decreased in the order of methanol, ethanol, and 2-propanol, as the solvent viscosity increased. The relative photolysis rates in hexane and cyclohexane, with respective relative viscosities of 0.33 and 1, were 1.5 and 1. There was no difference in the extent of the

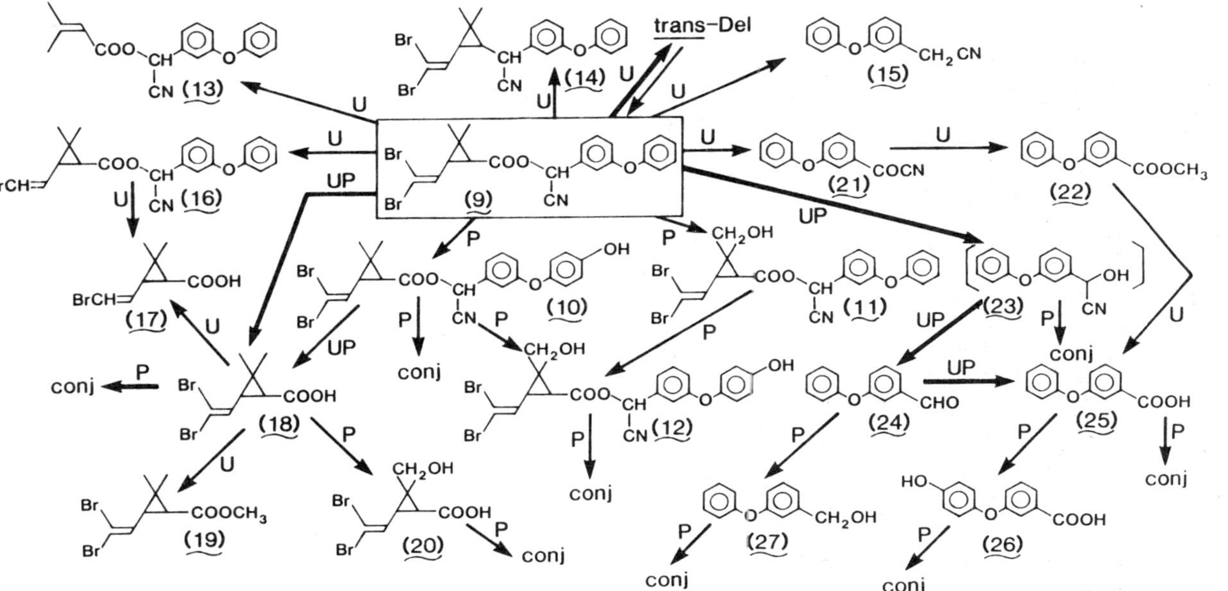


Figure 1. Degradation pathways of deltamethrin by UV light and in plants
U : UV light , P : plant (conj = sugar conjugate )

reaction on flushing the hexane with $O_2$ or $N_2$, while the triplet quenchers piperilene and 1,3-cyclohexadiene reduced the reaction rate in hexane.

At 30–50% conversion, the *trans*-[1R, 3S; αS] and -[1S, 3R; αS] isomers were the major photoproducts in aqueous acetonitrile, whereas they were observed in only minor amounts in methanol and were absent in hexane. The mono-debrominated esters (16) were the major ester products in methanol and hexane. The *cis*-acid (18) was always the major photoproduct from the acid moiety, with smaller amounts of the two isomeric debrominated acids (17).

Major products from the alcohol moiety were 3-phenoxybenzoic acid (25) (PBacid) in aqueous acetonitrile, 3-phenoxybenzyl cyanide (15) in hexane, and methyl 3-phenoxybenzoate (22) in methanol. Photolysis of 3-phenoxybenzoyl cyanide (21) gave methyl 3-phenoxybenzoate and the methyl ester of $Br_2CA$ (19) in methanol and PBacid in aqueous acetonitrile. Thus, it appears that the photoproducts obtained originated from cyclopropane ring opening and various recombinations, scission of the ester oxygen–benzyl carbon bond, scission of the acyl–oxygen bond, and/or reductive debromination (Ruzo et al., 1976, 1977).

A photodegradation study with $^{14}C$-deltamethrin in aqueous solution showed that such a solution, at pH 5, is hydrolytically stable. When exposed to simulated sunlight, degradation was induced. The primary product observed was PBacid. A half-life of 47.7 days was calculated for the non-sensitized system, but this was reduced to 4.03 days when sensitized with 1% acetone. Practically no volatile degradation products were observed (Bowman & Carpenter, 1987).

## 4.3 Environmental fate

The degradation and persistence of $^{14}C$-cyano- and $^{14}C$-phenoxy-deltamethrin was examined in a Dubbs fine sandy loam and a Memphis silt loam under aerobic laboratory conditions at 25 °C (Kaufman & Kayser 1979a); $^{14}C$-deltamethrin was applied at final concentrations equivalent to 0.02 and 0.2 kg/ha. Deltamethrin degradation occurred rapidly in both soils with 62–77%

and 52–60% of the $^{14}C$-cyano- and $^{14}C$-phenoxy-labels, respectively, being evolved as $^{14}CO_2$ during the 128-day incubation period. The half-life of deltamethrin varied from 11 to 19 days in the two soil types.

The effect of soil temperature on the degradation of deltamethrin was also examined in Dubbs fine sandy loam under laboratory conditions using $^{14}C$-cyano- and $^{14}C$-vinyl-labelled deltamethrin (Kaufman & Kayser 1979b). Degradation and evolution of $^{14}C$-labelled forms of deltamethrin occurred most rapidly at 25 °C and most slowly in soils incubated at 10 °C. The half-life of deltamethrin was 46, 13, and 27 days in soils incubated at 10, 25, and 40 °C, respectively.

The results of these two studies indicate that deltamethrin degradation occurs by two principal pathways (Fig. 2): hydrolysis of the ester linkage to yield $Br_2CA$ (18) and 3-phenoxybenzoic acid; and hydrolysis of the cyano group to yield first the amide, and subsequently the carboxylic acid (DCOOH) analogues of deltamethrin. $Br_2CA$ accumulated to a maximum of 5.7% of the original $^{14}C$ in soil incubated at 40 °C, whereas DCOOH accumulated at 10 °C (to a maximum of 5.3%). However, both products decreased in concentration by the end of the 64-day incubation period. In the first experiment, DCOOH was also identified as the major degradation product to reach a maximum concentration of 6–9% of the original $^{14}C$. But it ultimately dissipated to less than 2% at the end of the 128-day incubation period.

From the $^{14}C$-phenoxy label, 3-phenoxybenzoic acid (PBacid) was identified as the main degradation product resulting from hydrolysis of the ester bond. This product was further degraded to yield both 3-(2-hydroxyphenoxy)-benzoic acid and 3-(4-hydroxyphenoxy) benzoic acid. In this experiment, DCOOH was the only deltamethrin degradation product detected in excess of 3% of the original material applied.

Although essentially no radiolabel was detected in the leachate from soil columns treated with $^{14}C$-deltamethrin, PBacid produced by degradation of deltamethrin was fairly mobile in the soil columns (Kaufman et al., 1981).

The degradation pathways are proposed in Fig.2.

The degradation of deltamethrin was also examined under anaerobic conditions using $^{14}C$-cyano- , $^{14}C$-phenoxy- , and $^{14}C$-vinyl-labelled materials for the tests (Kaufman & Kayser, 1980). Under anaerobic conditions, $^{14}CO_2$ evolution varied according to the $^{14}C$ label position and the time of flooding. Generally, flooding reduced or initially inhibited the rate of $^{14}CO_2$ dissipation. However, after one month, $^{14}CO_2$ dissipation started again, which suggested the presence of a unique microbial flora. It was also shown that all three carboxylic acids that accumulate initially in flooded soils are subsequently further degraded. Some reduction of PBacid to 3-phenoxybenzyl alcohol (PBalc) was also observed in these flooded soils.

When deltamethrin was applied to a sandy clay loam soil at 17.5 g/ha in an indoor incubation study and in two field experiments, the half-lives of deltamethrin were found to be 4.9 and 6.9 weeks under indoor and field conditions, respectively (Hill, 1983). This difference in the rate of decrease in the residue was attributed to climatic effects.

This was further confirmed by Hill & Schaalje (1985) who pointed out a first-order dissipation, if degree-days above 0 °C rather than days was used as the independent variable, when deltamethrin was applied by pipette to soils. When deltamethrin was boom-sprayed, a biphasic first-order plot was observed. A two-compartment model that predicts an initial fast loss of residue followed by a slower first-order degradation gave a good fit of the data.

Chapman & Harris (1981) examined the relative persistence of five pyrethroids, permethrin, cypermethrin, deltamethrin, fenpropathrin, and fenvalerate, in sand and organic soil at 28 °C, under laboratory conditions. All of the insecticides (1 mg/kg) were degraded more rapidly in natural soils than in sterilized soils, suggesting the importance of microbial degradation. The rate of degradation under non-sterilized conditions decreased as follows: fenpropathrin > permethrin > cypermethrin > fenvalerate > deltamethrin. Amounts of approximately 52% and 74% of the deltamethrin applied were recovered from the sand and organic soil, respectively, 8 weeks after treatment.

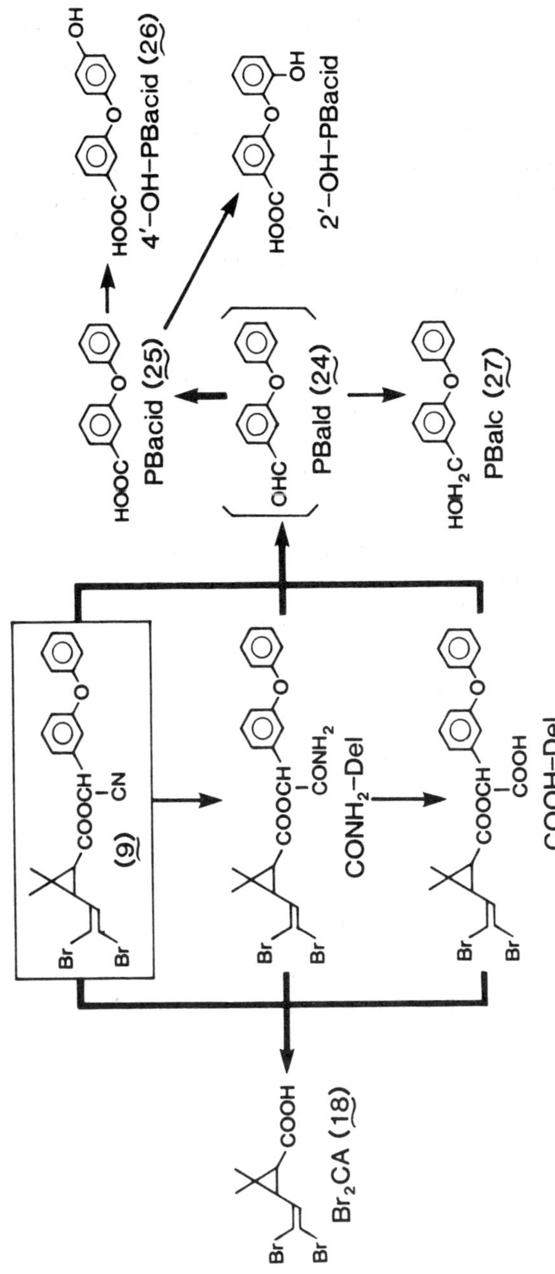


Figure 2. Degradation pathways of deltamethrin in soils

It was pointed out by Chapman et al. (1981) that biological processes played a major role in the degradation of deltamethrin in soils.

The degradation of deltamethrin was also investigated by Zhang et al. (1984) in an organic soil over a 180-day period. The half-life of deltamethrin was found to be 72 days, indicating that deltamethrin is likely to be less susceptible to degradation in organic soils than in mineral soils. Identification of metabolites present in the extractable phase confirmed the metabolic pathways previously reported by Kaufman. Levels of bound $^{14}C$ residues increased with the incubation period to reach 19% of the original $^{14}C$ after 180 days. Most of these bound $^{14}C$ residues were in the humic fraction. Bacterial and actinomycete populations increased in the treated soil, but fungal populations remained relatively stable during the incubation period.

The degradation of deltamethrin was also studied in two German soils. Half-lives for sandy soil and sandy loam soil were 35 and 60 days, respectively (Thier & Schmidt, 1977).

All these studies demonstrate that deltamethrin is readily and quickly degraded in the soil. The half-life of the compound depends on the nature of the soil as well as the temperature. Generally speaking, the half-life ranges from 11 to 72 days, under aerobic conditions. Deltamethrin degradation is slower under anaerobic or sterile conditions, indicating that microorganisms and other biological processes play a very important role.

The metabolism of deltamethrin in cotton plants was studied using material $^{14}C$-labelled at the dibromovinyl, benzylic, and cyano carbons. Under glasshouse conditions, the initial half-life of deltamethrin was 1.1 weeks and the time needed for 90% loss was 4.6 weeks. Conversion of deltamethrin to the *trans*-isomer occurred via photochemical reactions and, after 6 weeks, the *trans/cis* ratio was 0.44:1. Deltamethrin degraded more rapidly under field conditions to give a higher proportion of *trans*- to *cis*-isomers and large amounts of unextractable products. Trace amounts of three deltamethrin derivatives hydroxylated either at the 4′-position (10), or at the *trans* -methyl relative to the carboxy group in the acid moiety (7), or at both sites (12) were detected with all three $^{14}C$ preparations (Fig. 1). However, the major metabolites were free and conjugated $Br_2CA$ together with small quantities of the *trans*-hydroxymethyl derivatives (20) of $Br_2CA$ and 3-(4-hydroxyphenoxy) benzoic acid (26). The above compounds were analogues of those formed from permethrin and cypermethrin in plants. Several types of conjugated metabolites were isolated, but they were not fully characterized. One type was cleaved readily with β-glucosidase or hydrogen chloride to yield $Br_2CA$ and PBacid. Two other types were resistant to β-glucosidase, but cleaved readily with hydrogen chloride to yield $Br_2CA$ (from the dibromovinyl label) and 3-phenoxybenzoic acid, 3-phenoxybenzyl alcohol (from the alcohol label), and α-cyano-3-phenoxybenzyl alcohol (from the cyano and alcohol labels). The metabolites of deltamethrin identified in plants were analogous to those in mammals, except for the conjugated products.

The metabolism of deltamethrin and its degradation products in cotton and bean leaf disks has also been studied. Limited conversion (approximately 6%) of deltamethrin occurred to give $Br_2CA$ and 3-phenoxybenzyl alcohol (27) (PBalc) conjugates. The ester cleavage products used as substrates underwent more extensive metabolism, and two to three types of glucosides were formed from $Br_2CA$ and four from PBalc. 3-Phenoxybenzaldehyde (24), administered directly or as the cyanohydrin (23), was reduced to PBalc, though part was oxidized to PBacid (Ruzo & Casida, 1979).

## 4.4 Bioaccumulation

Bioaccumulation studies with fish have shown that pyrethroids have bioconcentration factors (BCFs) that are far lower than those predicted from the correlation between the $K_{ow}$ partition coefficient and BCF. The low accumulation can be attributed to metabolism by the fish and to the reduced bioavailability to fish of deltamethrin bound by dissolved organic carbon and suspended colloids. Metabolic kinetics were assessed by Cary (1978) in *Ictalurus punctatus* maintained for 30 days in the water of a hydrosoil system, in which the soil was treated with a dose of 125 g a.i./ha (10 times the normal agricultural dose) and then flooded after 31 days. During the exposure period, none of the 300 fish died or behaved abnormally despite a final deltamethrin concentration of 2.19 μg/litre, which is more than 3 times the acute 96-h $LC_{50}$ of 0.63 μg/litre (Table 6). During a third phase, fish were introduced into an uncontaminated liquid medium, continuously renewed, to monitor elimination of deltamethrin or its metabolites. The main results are given in Table 5.

Table 5. Bioaccumulation factors after exposure of *Ictalurus punctatus* and depuration kinetics[a]

| Organ | Value of bioconcentration factor (BCF)[b] during exposure, 30 days | $^{14}C$ elimination (%) after depuration of | |
|---|---|---|---|
| | | 1 day | 14 days |
| muscles | 25 | <50 | 77 |
| viscera | 972 | 67 | 86 |
| carcasses | 41 | >50 | 93 |
| body as a whole | 144 | >50 | 93 |

[a] From: Cary (1978).
[b] BCF : μg/kg concentration in fish/μg/litre concentration in water.

Muir et al. (1985) monitored the fate and uptake of $^{14}C$-labelled deltamethrin in organisms in experimental ponds over 306 days. Initial concentrations of the pyrethroid ranged from 1.8 to 2.5 μg/litre. The deltamethrin rapidly became distributed in suspended solids, plants, sediment, and air with a half-life of 2–4 h in the water. Aquatic plants (the floating duckweed *Lemna* sp. and a submerged/floating weed (*Potomageton berchtoldi*) accumulated deltamethrin at concentrations of between 253 and 1021 μg/kg, respectively, 24 h after treatment, but the compound had all disappeared within 14 days. Fathead minnows, *Pimephales promelas,* showed bioconcentration factors of 248–907. Although radioactivity remained in the fish throughout the experimental period, presumably in the fat, the levels fell steadily and no effects were seen on the fish.

# 5. KINETICS AND METABOLISM

## 5.1 Metabolism in experimental animals

Metabolic pathways of deltamethrin in mammals are summarized in Fig. 3.

After oral administration to male rats at 0.64–1.60 mg/kg, the acid and alcohol moieties of deltamethrin were almost completely eliminated from the body within 2–4 days (Ruzo et al., 1978). On the other hand, the cyano group was eliminated more slowly, the total recovery during 8 days being 79% of the radiocarbon dose (43% and 36% in the urine and faeces, respectively). Tissue residues of deltamethrin labelled with $^{14}C$ at the dibromovinyl carbon in the acid moiety and the benzylic carbon in the alcohol moiety were generally very low, whereas residue levels in the fat were somewhat higher (0.1–0.2 mg/kg). Residue levels of the radiocarbon derived from the cyano group were relatively high, especially in the skin and stomach. Essentially, all the radiocarbon in the stomach was thiocyanate. No noticeable $^{14}CO_2$ was evolved from any of the radioactive preparations, including the CN-labelled group, in contrast to the CN group from fenvalerate, which yielded $^{14}CO_2$ in considerable amounts.

The major metabolic reactions of deltamethrin were oxidation (at the *trans* methyl relative to carbonyl group of the acid moiety and at the 2′-, 4′-, and 5-positions of the alcohol moiety), cleavage of the ester linkage, and conversion of the cyano portion to thiocyanate and 2-iminothiazolidine-4-carboxylic acid (31) (ITCA) (see Fig. 3). These carboxylic acid and phenol derivatives were conjugated with sulfuric acid, glycine, and/or glucuronic acid.

The major faecal metabolites were unchanged deltamethrin (9), accounting for 13–21% of the dose, followed by 4′-OH-(10) and 5-OH-deltamethrin (28), and a trace amount of 2′-OH-deltamethrin (29). Intact deltamethrin and the 4′-OH-derivative appeared not only as the administered S-epimer, but also in parts as the R-epimer, probably due to artefactural racemization on

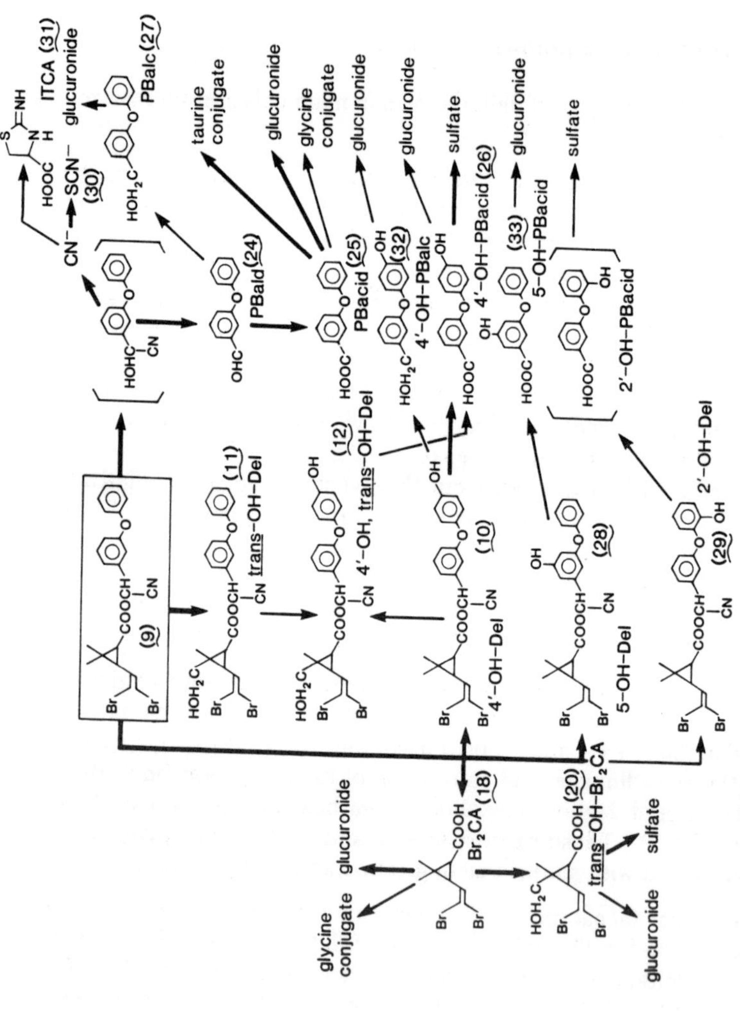


Figure 3. Metabolic pathways of deltamethrin in mammals

exchange of the α-position hydrogen in methanol solution. The metabolites from the acid moiety were mostly 3-(2,2-dibromovinyl)-2,2-dimethylcyclopropanecarboxylic acid (18) ($Br_2CA$) in free form (10% of the dose), glucuronide (51%) and glycine (trace level) conjugates, and OH-$Br_2CA$(20) in free form and glucuronide conjugate ($<1\%$).

The major metabolites of the aromatic portion of the alcohol moiety were 3-phenoxybenzoic acid (25) (PBacid) in free form (5%), and glucuronide (13%) and glycine (4%) conjugates and its 4′-hydroxy derivative (26) (4′-OH-PBacid).

Sulfate of 4′-OH-PBacid accounted for about 50% of the dose, together with small amounts of free (4%) and glucuronide forms (2%). The CN group was converted mainly to thiocyanate (30) and, in small amounts, to ITCA (31) (Ruzo et al., 1978). The *trans*-isomer of deltamethrin was also rapidly metabolized and yielded almost the same metabolites as deltamethrin, though 5-OH-derivative was found in the *cis*-isomer, but not in the *trans*-isomer (Ruzo et al., 1978).

When a single oral dose of $^{14}C$-(acid-, alcohol-, or cyano-labelled) deltamethrin was administered to male mice at 1.7–4.4 mg/kg, the acid moiety and the aromatic portion of the alcohol moiety were rapidly and almost completely excreted, whereas the CN group was excreted relatively slowly (Ruzo et al., 1979).

Gray & Rickard (1982) followed the distribution of $^{14}C$-acid- , $^{14}C$-alcohol- , and $^{14}C$-cyano-labelled deltamethrin and selected metabolites in the liver, blood, cerebrum, cerebellum, and spinal cord after iv administration of a toxic, but non-lethal, dose (1.75 mg/kg) to rats. Approximately 50% of the dose was cleared from the blood within 0.7–0.8 min, after which the rate of clearance decreased. 3-Phenoxybenzoic acid (PBacid) was isolated from the blood *in vivo*, and was also the major metabolite when $^{14}C$-alcohol-labelled deltamethrin was incubated with blood *in vitro*. Deltamethrin levels in the liver peaked at 7–10 nmol/g at 5 min and then decreased to 1 nmol/g by 30 min. In contrast, peak central nervous system levels of deltamethrin were achieved within 1 min (0.5 nmol/g), decreasing to 0.2 nmol/g at 15 min, and remaining stable until 60 min. Peak levels of deltamethrin were not related to the severity of toxicity, though the levels of unextractable pentane radiolabel did appear to be correlated with signs of motor toxicity. Experiments with brain homogenates from animals injected iv with deltamethrin failed to reproduce the pentane-unextractable radioactivity *in vitro* and metabolism of the compound was not demonstrated.

The major metabolic pathways of deltamethrin in mice were similar to those in rats, though there were some differences. These included the presence of more unchanged deltamethrin in mouse faeces than in rat faeces. In mouse faeces, there were 4 monohydroxy ester metabolites (2′-OH- , 4′-OH- , 5-OH- , and *trans*-OH-deltamethrin (11)) and one dihydroxy metabolite (12) (4′-OH-*trans*-OH-deltamethrin) that were not found in mouse urine. Major metabolites from the acid moiety in mice were $Br_2CA$, *trans*-OH-$Br_2CA$ (20), and their glucuronide and sulfate conjugates. Among them, *trans*-OH-$Br_2CA$-sulfate was detected only in mice, but not in rats. Compared with rats, much larger amounts of *trans*-OH-$Br_2CA$ and its conjugates were formed in mice. A major metabolite of the alcohol moiety in mice was the taurine conjugate of PBacid in the urine, which was not detected in rats. Generally, mice produced smaller amounts of phenolic compounds compared with rats. Also, 3-phenoxybenzaldehyde (24) (PBald), 3-phenoxybenzyl alcohol (32) (PBalc), and its glucuronide, and glucuronides of 3-(4-hydroxyphenoxy)benzyl alcohol (33) (4′-OH-PBalc) and 5-hydroxy-3-phenoxybenzoic acid (34) (5-OH-PBacid) were found in mice, but not in rats. When mice were given an ip dose of $^{14}C$-deltamethrin, with or without piperonyl butoxide (PBO) and/or *S,S,S*-tributylphosphorotrithioate (DEF), the same metabolites were obtained as with oral administration. However, DEF decreased the hydrolytic products relative to the controls, while PBO decreased the oxidation products (Ruzo et al., 1979).

The comparison between the excreted radioactivity of $^{14}C$-deltamethrin in rats treated by the percutaneous route and iv (controls) showed that only 3.6% of the dosage applied on the skin was absorbed and excreted in 24 h with 1.1% excreted during the first 6 h. Since the rat skin is more permeable than human skin, the uptake of deltamethrin through the human skin should be relatively weak (Pottier et al., 1982).

## 5.2 Metabolism and fate in farm animals

In a metabolic study, $^{14}C$-deltamethrin was administered orally to lactating dairy cows at the rate of 10 mg/kg body weight per day for 3 consecutive days. It was poorly absorbed and mainly eliminated in the faeces as unchanged deltamethrin. Only 4–6% of the administered $^{14}C$ was eliminated in the urine, and 0.42–1.62% was secreted in the milk. The radiocarbon contents of various tissues were generally very low with the exception of those of the liver, kidney, and fat, which were higher (Akhtar et al. 1986). Deltamethrin degradation occurred by cleavage of the ester bond, as already reported in rats and mice (Ruzo et al. 1978, 1979). The enzymes responsible for the ester bond cleavage were located in cow liver homogenate, mainly in the microsomal fraction, as seen in an *in vitro* study (Akhtar, 1984). Metabolites resulting from ester bond cleavage were further metabolized and/or conjugated, resulting in a large number of compounds excreted in the urine (see Fig. 3). In milk, the major identifiable radiolabelled compound was deltamethrin.

In a feeding study by Akhtar et al. (1987), deltamethrin was administered twice daily to lactating dairy cows in portions of their daily feed at the rate of 2 or 10 mg/kg diet for 28 consecutive days. The level of 2 mg/kg diet was the residue level found in a recently treated pasture (Hill & Johnson, 1987), whereas 10 mg/kg diet was five times this level. Deltamethrin residues in the milk were dose-dependent and appeared to reach a plateau between 7 and 9 days after the start of treatment. At the high deltamethrin intake of 10 mg/kg diet, the deltamethrin residue in milk was about 0.025 mg/litre. Deltamethrin residues in tissues were measured 1, 4, and 9 days after the last dose. At the 10 mg/kg diet intake, very small amounts of deltamethrin residues were found in the liver (< 0.005 mg/kg), kidney (< 0.002 mg/kg), and muscle (0.002–0.014 mg/kg). Residues in fat were about 0.04 mg/kg and 0.2 mg/kg for the 2 and 10 mg/kg intake, respectively. Depletion of deltamethrin residues in milk was very rapid (estimated half-life was about 1 day); while in fat (renal and subcutaneous) the half-life was 7–9 days. $Br_2CA$ (3-(2,2-dibromovinyl)-2,2-dimethylcyclopropanecarboxylic acid) and PBacid (3-phenoxybenzoic acid) were the only metabolites detected in the milk and tissues of treated cows. In all cases, they were found at trace levels of < 0.0235 mg/litre and < 0.034 mg/litre, respectively. These two metabolites were also previously identified in rats and mice as the major degradation products of deltamethrin (Ruzo et al., 1978, 1979).

The fate of $^{14}C$-deltamethrin was examined in Leghorn hens (Akhtar et al., 1985). When laying hens were administered 7.5 mg of $^{14}C$-labelled deltamethrin/hen per day orally for 3 consecutive days, about 83% and 90% of the administered $^{14}C$ was eliminated during the first 24 h and 48 h after dosing, respectively. Tissue residues were generally very low with the exception of those in the liver and kidney. Very low levels of residues were found in eggs obtained within the first 24 h after dosing, but levels increased reaching a peak within 48 h of the last dose. Residue levels were higher in the yolk (up to 0.6 mg/kg) than in the albumen (up to 0.2 mg/kg), which is probably related to the lipid content of yolks. Metabolites were the same as those found in rats and mice.

These studies showed that feeding domestic animals on deltamethrin-treated feed resulted in very low levels of residues (if any) in products of animal origin and is unlikely to present a hazard for the consumer.

## 5.3 Enzymatic systems for biotransformation

Deltamethrin (1 μg) was incubated at 37 °C for 30 min with each of the following mouse microsome preparations; *a*) tetraethyl pyrophosphate (TEPP)-treated microsomes (no esterase and oxidase activity); *b*) normal microsomes (esterase activity); *c*) TEPP-treated microsomes plus NADPH (oxidase activity); and *d*) normal microsomes plus NADPH (esterase plus oxidase activity) (Shono et al., 1979). Deltamethrin was more rapidly metabolized under the oxidase system than under the esterase system. The major site of ring hydroxylation was the 4′-position and the secondary site was the 5-position. The *trans* methyl group was an important site of hydroxylation of the esters and *cis* methyl oxidation was evident in the metabolites of the cleaved acid moiety. The preferred sites of hydroxylation were as follows; *trans* of dimethyl group, 4′-position in the phenol group, and *cis* of the dimethyl group, which was equal to the 5-position in the phenoxy group. Cleavage of deltamethrin to cyanohydrin may result from both esterase and oxidase enzyme activities, since larger amounts of the cleaved products were evident in the oxidase system.

However, at a much higher (approximately 35-fold) concentration of deltamethrin than that in the above study, it was not detectably hydrolysed (Miyamoto, 1976; Soderlund & Casida, 1977).

Deltamethrin was hydrolysed by esterases in the blood, brain, kidney, and stomach of mice yielding PBald and PBacid (Ruzo et al., 1979).

## 5.4 Metabolism in human beings

Three young male human volunteers underwent a complete medical check-up one week prior to the morning of the study. Each of them received a single dose of 3 mg of $^{14}C$-deltamethrin mixed in 1 g glucose and diluted first in 10 ml PEG 300 and again in 150 ml water. Total radioactivity was 1.8 ± 0.09 mBq. Samples of blood, urine, saliva, and faeces were taken at intervals over 5 days. Clinical and biological examinations were performed every 12 h during the trial and one week after its termination. Radioactivity in the biological samples was measured with a liquid scintillation spectrometer. The clinical and biological checks did not detect any abnormal findings. There were no signs of side effects or intolerance reactions, either during or after the trial period. The maximum plasma radioactivity appeared between 1 and 2 h after administration of the product, and remained over the detection limit (0.2 KBq/litre) during the 48 h. The apparent elimination half-life was between 10.0 and 11.5 h. The radioactivity of blood cells, as well as the saliva, was extremely low. Urinary excretion was 51–59% of the initial radioactivity; 90% of this radioactivity was excreted during the 24 h following absorption. The apparent half-life of urinary excretion was 10.0–13.5 h, which is consistent with the plasma data. Faecal elimination at the end of the observation period represented 10–26% of the dose. The total faecal plus urine elimination was around 64–77% of the initial dose after 96 h (Papalexiou et al., 1984).

# 6. EFFECTS ON ORGANISMS IN THE ENVIRONMENT

## 6.1 Aquatic organisms

### 6.1.1 *Acute toxicity for fish*

Acute toxicity data for deltamethrin in fish have been summarized by L'Hotellier & Vincent (1986) (Table 6). From this, it appears that deltamethrin is highly toxic for fish, though the toxicity varies with the formulation tested.

Zitko et al. (1979) established a 96-h lethal threshold for Atlantic salmon (*Salmo salar*) of 1.97 μg/litre.

Table 6. Acute toxicity of deltamethrin tested as the technical or formulated product on fish; lethal concentrations all expressed as μg active ingredient (a.i.)/litre (96-h)

| Species (Common name) | System[a] | $LC_{50}$ (μg/litre) tested as technical product | Ref. No. | $LC_{50}$ (μg/litre) tested as formulated product[b] | Ref. No. |
|---|---|---|---|---|---|
| *Alburnus alburnus* (Bleak) | S | 0.69 | 4 | 82 (ULV) | 4 |
| *Brachydanio rerio* (Zebra fish) | F,S | 2.0 | 10 | - | |
| *Cyprinodon macularius* (Desert pupfish) | S | - | | 0.6[c] (EC) | 13 |
| *Cyprinodon variegatus*[d] (Sheepshead minnow) | S | - | | 0.9 (EC) | 19 |
| *Cyrpinus carpio* (Common carp) | F, S | 1.84<br>0.86 | 4<br>3 | 0.65 (EC)<br>210.0 (ULV) | 4 |
| *Gambusia affinis* (Mosquito fish) | F, S | - | | 1.0[c] (EC) | 13 |
| *Ictalurus nebulosus* (Brown bullhead) | F, S | 1.2 | 7 | 2.3 (EC) | 15 |
| *Ictalurus punctatus* (Hannel catfish) | F, S | 0.63 | 8 | - | |

Table 6 (*continued*)

| Species (Common name) | System[a] | $LC_{50}$ (μg/litre) tested as technical product | Ref. No. | $LC_{50}$ (μg/litre) tested as formulated product[b] | | Ref. No. |
|---|---|---|---|---|---|---|
| *Idus idus melanotus* (Golden orfe) | S | - | | 1.2 | (EC) | 16 |
| *Lebistes reticulatus* (Guppy) | F, S | - | | 1.8 | (EC) | 17 |
| *Lepomis gibbosus* (Pumpkinseed sunfish) | F, S | 0.58 | 5 | 0.87 | (EC) | 14 |
| *Lepomis machrochirus* (Bluegill sunfish) | F | 1.2 | 6 | - | | |
| *Osteochilus hasselti*[e] (Nilem carp) | S | - | | 1.2 | (EC) | 20 |
| *Puntius gonionotus*[e] (Jawa carp) | F,S | - | | 0.87 | (EC) | 18 |
| *Rhodeus sericeus amarus* | S | 1.12 | 4 | 140 | (ULV) | 4 |
| *Salmo gairdneri* (Rainbow trout) | F, S | 0.39 | 1 | 2.2 | (EC) | 12 |
| *Salmo salar* | | 1.97 | 2 | 0.59 | (EC) | 2 |
| *Salmo trutta* (Brown trout) | F, S | - | | 4.7[c] | (EC) | 11 |
| *Sarotherodon* mossambicus[e] | F, S | 3.5 | 9 | 2.0 | (EC) | 9 |
| *Tilapia mossambica*[e] | F, S | - | | 0.8[c] | (EC) | 13 |

[a] F: Flow system, S: Static condition.
[b] EC: 25 g a.i./litre; ULV: l g a.i./litre; values in a.i. equivalent obtained by calculation.
[c] $LC_{50}$ (48-h)
[d] Marine fish.
[e] River or pond fish from tropical areas (water temperature ≥24 °C).

*References*

(1) Knauf & Horlein (1979); (2) Zitko et al. (1979); (3) Knauf & Schulze(1977a); (4) Gulyas & Csanyi (undated); (5) Waltersdorfer & Schulze (1976a); (6) Buccafusco et al. (1977a); (7) Knauf & Schulze (1977b); (8) Buccafusco et al. (1977b); (9) Adeney et al. (1980); (10) Lepailleur & Chambon (1984); (11) Lhoste et al. (1979); (12) Waltersdorfer & Schulze (1976c); (13) Mulla et al (1978); (14) Waltersdorfer & Schulze (1976d); (15) Knauf & Schulze (1977b); (16) Waltersdorfer & Schulze (1976b); (17) Waltersdorfer & Schulze (1976a); (18) Santosa & Hadi (1980); (19) Heitmuller et al, (1978); (20) Santosa (1983)

### 6.1.2 Acute toxicity for other aquatic organisms

Data on aquatic organisms other than fish are presented in Table 7 and are of the same order as those for fish, although the oyster (*Crassostrea virginica*) is somewhat more tolerant and the Northern lobster (*Homarus americanus*) (96-h lethal threshold 0.0014 μg/litre) is far more sensitive (Zitko et al., 1979).

Mohsen & Mulla (1981) exposed aquatic insect larvae to deltamethrin (as a 2.5% emulsifiable concentrate) for 1 h under flow-through conditions, and calculated the $LC_{50}$ after a 24-h holding period. For the target species blackfly (*Simulium virgatum*) an $LC_{50}$ of 0.9 μg/litre was calculated. Non-target species tested, mayfly (*Baetis parvus*) and caddisfly (*Hydropsyche californica*), were found to be more susceptible, with $LC_{50}$ values of 0.4 μg/litre.

Table 7. Acute toxicity of deltamethrin tested as technical or formulated product on other aquatic organisms—lethal concentrations expressed as μg active ingredient (a.i.)/litre (96-h)[a]

| Species | $LC_{50}$ (μg/litre) tested as technical product | $LC_{50}$ (μg/litre) tested as formulated product[b] |
|---|---|---|
| *Crassostrea virginica* (Eastern oyster) | - | 12.0 |
| *Daphnia magna* (Water flea) | 5[c] | - |
| *Gammarus pulex* (Scud) | - | 0.03[c] |
| *Penaeus duorarum* (Pink shrimp) | - | 0.35 |
| *Uca pugilatorulosus* (Fiddler crab) | - | 1.1 |
| *Bufo bufo* (larvae) (Common toad) | - | 0.93 |

[a] Adapted from: L'Hotellier & Vincent (1986).
[b] EC: 25 g a.i./litre; ULV: l g a.i./litre; values in a.i. equivalent obtained by calculation.
[c] $LC_{50}$ (48-h).

Table 8. Acute toxicity[a] of deltamethrin formulation[b] in freshwater mussels, under static conditions at 21–23 °C[c]

| Species | 24-h | 48-h | 72-h | 96-h | 7-day |
|---|---|---|---|---|---|
| *Anodonta cygnea* | nd | nd | ~24.6 | 12.0 | 7.6 |
| *Anodonta anatina* | nd | nd | nd | ~23.4 | 10.3 |
| *Unio pictorum* | nd | ~31.8 | 9.7 | 7.0 | 6.0 |

[a] $LC_{50}$ μg active ingredient (a.i.)/litre): values in a.i. equivalent obtained by calculation..
[b] ULV 0.12%.
[c] From: Varanka (1987).

Varanka (1987) investigated the effects of deltamethrin on three species of freshwater mussels. Results presented in Table 8 show that the mussels are very insensitive to the pyrethroid.

### 6.1.3 *Field studies and community effects*

Two experimental pond studies have been performed. Tooby et al. (1981) reported that application of deltamethrin to static water at 10 g a.i./ha did not have any lethal effects on two fish species (*Canassius auratus*, *Rutilus rutilus*) or on molluscs. Aquatic insects and crustaceans present were killed. Rawn et al. (1985) applied deltamethrin at a similar rate and also reported that no fish were killed. The half-life of deltamethrin in the pond was 2–4 h for water and 2–14 days for bottom sediment.

Neto et al. (1983) sprayed-flooded fields in Brazil, at intervals of 2 days, with rates of deltamethrin progressively increased at 5, 10, 12, and 13 g a.i./ha. The expected concentrations in water from these applications were between 3 and 7 μg/litre. No mortality was recorded in fish placed in the sprayed area in experimental cages. Slight "agitation" was reported after exposure to the highest dose.

Impact assessments on the use of deltamethrin on paddy fields have been made in the field in various countries throughout the world. The maximum normal usage rate of the compound was 6.5 g a.i./ha. In these studies, fish (*Tilapia* spp., *Cyprinus carpio, Gambusia* spp.) tolerated deltamethrin up to 18.75 g a.i./ha without any adverse effects. The compound is known to be toxic for aquatic organisms and is not recommended for use over water under any but exceptional circumstances. However, it has been used to control vectors of major human diseases, i.e., mosquitos and blackfly (*Elossina* spp.), where benefit outweighed potential risk. In these cases, extensive field evaluations of the environmental impact have been made. While there have not been any instances of fish kills from these applications, there are reports of large numbers of deaths of aquatic invertebrates. The populations usually recovered rapidly and all studies have shown numbers back to normal before the compound was applied again in the following season. It is suggested that relatively resistant parts of the population soon recolonize the area; immigration also occurs (Takken et al., 1978; Smies et al., 1980; Baldry et al., 1981; Everts et al., 1983).

### 6.1.4 *Appraisal*

Notwithstanding its high toxicity for fish and crustacea, the results of many studies, as well as the wide use of deltamethrin for several years, have confirmed that its normal use does not cause significant mortality in fish populations. This difference is due to its strong adsorption on soil and its rapid breakdown, decreasing its bioavailability under field conditions.

## 6.2 Terrestrial organisms

### 6.2.1 *Plants*

Hargreaves & Cooper (1979) sprayed glasshouse-grown tomato seedlings with 50 mg deltamethrin/litre (2.5% emulsifiable concentrate) 3 weeks after emergence and again 7 days later. Three days after the second application, plants were examined for damage. No damage was found and, at this rate of use, deltamethrin was not phytotoxic.

### 6.2.2 *Soil microorganisms*

In a study by Tu (1980) on the effects of 5 pyrethroids on microbial populations and their activity in soil, 0.5 mg deltamethrin/kg incorporated into sandy loams (residues under normal use conditions would be of the order of < 0.001 mg/kg) produced only a few transient effects. No effects were noted on the nitrifying microorganisms and their capacity to produce nitrate and there were no inhibitory effects on deshydrogenase or urease activity. Deltamethrin induced an increase in oxygen consumption because of an increase in microbial respiration (probably linked with the microbial degradation of deltamethrin). It also stimulated the growth of soil fungi and inhibited the development of bacteria. Four weeks after treatment, deltamethrin-treated soil recovered completely and microorganism activity was equal to that in untreated soil.

### 6.2.3 *Soil fauna*

#### 6.2.3.1 *Earthworms*

When deltamethrin at 12.5 g a.i./ha (high agricultural dose) was incorporated into the soil to a depth of 1 cm, there were no toxic effects on earthworms *(Lumbricus terrestris)* during an observation period of 28 days (Bouche & Fayolle, 1979). However, significant toxic effects on earthworms were observed at levels of 60–125 g a.i./ha (5–10 times the highest rates applied in agriculture).

In another study with *Eisenia foetida andrei*, deltamethrin incorporated in artificial soil at concentrations of 1.7 mg/kg and 10 mg/kg did not produce any lethal effects (Chambon & Lepailleur, 1984).

#### 6.2.3.2 *Slugs*

Lettuce leaves treated with 4 times normal dosage rates, were fed to slugs (*Agrolimax* sp.). Leaves were quickly consumed but no toxic effects (mortality or activity) were observed (Ricou, 1978).

### 6.2.3.3 Soil arthropods

Under laboratory conditions, deltamethrin, applied topically and by immersion, was very toxic for the carabid beetle *Pterostichus. melanarius* (Illiger). Under natural conditions in the field, deltamethrin applied at normal dose rates was not toxic for these organisms (Dunning et al., 1981).

Everts et al. (1985) monitored the effects, on non-target organisms, of various compounds when used for the control of tsetse fly in the Ivory Coast in Africa. Deltamethrin was the most effective compound against the tsetse and also killed non-target musca flies. After deltamethrin spraying, Orthoptera and Procto- trupoidea were also significantly decreased while Nematocera increased in number. The results of this study suggest that ground spraying of the pyrethroid had greater effects on terrestrial arthropods than aerial applications.

Concurrent laboratory and field studies were conducted on the effects of deltamethrin on beneficial predatory spiders in a polder area of the Netherlands (Everts et al., 1988). During two growing seasons, 2800 samples were taken over an area of 17 different fields. The authors found that effects on spiders were eliminated when it rained soon after application, since the effect of the pyrethroid appeared to be indirect, causing the dehydration of spiders. This different response under dry and damp conditions was confirmed in the laboratory. However, reduction of spider numbers in the field was much greater than predicted from laboratory tests and recovery was more rapid in laboratory populations than in field populations. The uptake and effects of deltamethrin were greater through exposure to residues than through contact or oral exposure. There was a positive correlation between temperature and the toxicity of deltamethrin for spiders in the field. This contrasted with reports of a negative correlation for target insects reported in the literature. Laboratory studies showed that the negative temperature effect only occurred when spiders could not drink. It appeared that qualitative prediction from laboratory to field was possible but that quantitative prediction was not.

### 6.2.4 Beneficial insects

#### 6.2.4.1 Honey-bees

Single applications of deltamethrin are highly toxic for honey-bees (*Apis mellifera*). Stevenson et al (1978) found a contact $LD_{50}$ of 0.051 µg/bee and an oral $LD_{50}$ of 0.079 µg/bee.

Arzone & Vidano (1978) did not find any difference in mortality between controls and bees fed on sugar solutions containing 0.2 µg deltamethrin/litre. Increased mortality was recorded at all higher exposures reaching 100 % within 1 h at a concentration of 12.5 µg/litre.

In the field, direct treatment of caged bees caused a high mortality rate with doses of from 11.2 g/ha upwards (Atkins et al., 1976). Rape flowers were treated at a rate of 0.75 g a.i./100 litre and 1.5 g a.i./100 litre with an emulsifiable concentrate formulation, 25 g/litre; control plots were treated with water. Cages (3×2×2 m) containing a small hive (2 frames + open brood) were put over the treated flowers once the spray had dried. The mortality of the bees was then assessed over 7 days. The average mortalities were not significantly higher in the treated plots than in water-sprayed control plots (Louveaux et al., 1977).

However, Bocquet et al. (1980, 1983) demonstrated, after 3 years of field experiments, that deltamethrin under field conditions was innocuous at doses up to 12.5 g/ha. They also noted a repellant effect by the formulating materials, which lasted for 2–3 h. Further studies have been reported by Florelli et al. (1987a,b).

#### 6.2.4.2 Foliar insects

Deltamethrin was 70 times more toxic to the tobacco budworm (*Heliothis virescens*) than to its predator, green lacewing (*Chrysopa carnea*), but it was only 1.25 times more toxic to the tobacco budworm than to its parasite (*Campoletis sonorensis*) (Plapp & Bull, 1978).

In an apple orchard, where deltamethrin was applied at 12.5 mg/kg, no predatory mites (*Typhlodromus pyri*) were found during 10 weeks of observation, but spider mites (*Paponychus ulmi*) were not affected. The elimination of the predatory mite led to a marked increase in spider mite populations, later in the same season (Aliniazee & Cranham, 1980).

The impact of deltamethrin used against the English grain aphid (*Sitobion avenae*) was studied in 1983, 1984, and 1985 in the Paris basin. This study was carried out on wheat with pitfall traps, yellow water traps, suction sampling (D-vac), and sampling of ears. Effects were noted on: *S. avenae*, phytophagous Diptera (*Opimyza florum, Phytomyza nigra,* and *Oscinella frit*), Homoptera (*Zyginidia scutellaris, Metopolophium dirhodum*), Thysanoptera (*Limothrips cerealium, Acolothrips intermedius*), predatory Diptera (Empididae, Dolichopodidae), and on spiders (Erigonidae, Lycosidae, Linyphiidae, Theridiidae). The detritiphagous insects (Sciaridae, Chironomidae), the Carabidae and Staphylinidae and most microhymenoptera showed little or no difference after treatment. During the 3 years, no differences were observed from year to year as a result of field treatment, populations appearing homogeneous at the beginning of each trial (Fischer & Chambon, 1987).

A large-scale field trial was carried out in 1984 in southern England to investigate the side-effects of deltamethrin on non-target arthropods in winter wheat. The insecticides were applied in June and two methods, suction sampling (D-vac) and quadrats, were used to sample the arthropods for up to 75 days after treatment. During the post-treatment period, the numbers of Carabidae and Staphylinidae adults found in D-vac samples were reduced by 22% and 20%, respectively, compared with the controls (Vickerman et al., 1987a).

In the same field trial, arthropods were sampled with a D-vac for 11 weeks. Total numbers were similar in the control and deltamethrin-treated plots. The numbers of Empididae were reduced by deltamethrin, but Dolichopodidae were more numerous in treated than in control plots. The numbers of *Aphidius* spp. were higher in the deltamethrin-treated plots than in the control plots. The numbers of Coccinellidae larvae were reduced (Vickerman et al., 1987b).

### 6.2.5 Birds

#### 6.2.5.1 Laboratory studies

Data on the acute toxicity of deltamethrin for birds are given in Table 9.

The toxicity of deltamethrin for birds is very low. Both technical grade and commercially formulated deltamethrin administered in feed at 100 mg/kg diet was not palatable to Japanese quail (*Coturnix coturnix japonica*), with strong individual variations. Unpalatability diminished after repeated exposure and even became reversed in the case of the purified deltamethrin, which attracted quail already suffering from toxic effects (David, 1981).

Groups of 39 female Japanese quail (*Coturnix coturnix japonica*) were given daily doses of 0, 0.2, or 1 mg technical deltamethrin per animal, by gavage, over 34 days. No significant effects were observed on reproduction (De Lavaur et al., 1985).

Table 9. Acute toxicity of deltamethrin for birds

| Species | Sex | Application | $LD_{50}$ (mg/kg) | Reference |
|---|---|---|---|---|
| Red partridge (*Alectonis tufa*) | male & female | oral | >3000 | Grolleau & Giban, 1976b |
| Grey partridge (*Perdix perdix*) | male & female | oral | >1800 | Grolleau & Griban, 1976b |
| Chicken (*Gallus domestica*) | | oral | >1000 | Grandadam, 1976 |
| Hen | adult female | oral | >2500 | Ross et al, 1978 |
| Mallard duck (*Anas platyrhynchos*) | | oral | >4640 | Beavers & Fink, 1977a |
| Game duck | | oral | >4000 | Grolleau & Griban, 1976a |

### 6.2.5.2 *Field studies on birds*

The low toxicity of deltamethrin for birds, indicated by laboratory studies, has been confirmed in the field. In studies on the ecological consequences of the use of the compound to control tsetse fly (Takken et al., 1978) and blackfly (Smies et al., 1980) in West Africa, populations of various species of insectivorous, granivorous, and piscivorous birds were examined before and after spraying. There were no indications of any effects on either numbers or species diversity.

# 7. EFFECTS ON EXPERIMENTAL ANIMALS AND *IN VITRO* TEST SYSTEMS

## 7.1 Single exposures

Tables 10 and 11 show the results of acute toxicity studies on various animal species. From these tables, it is clear that the vehicle has a great influence on the $LD_{50}$, probably by influencing absorption. Powder formulations and aqueous suspensions are significantly less toxic than formulations in oils or organic solvents (Pham Huu Chanh et al., 1984).

The acute oral toxicity of deltamethrin for rats produced such symptoms as: staining of the fur, excessive grooming, salivation, diarrhoea, drowsiness, weakness, dyspnoea, piloerection, ptosis, difficulty in walking, general motor incoordination, hypotonia, choreoathetosis, clonic seizures, and death (Glomot, 1979; Glomot et al., 1979, 1981a; Kavlock et al., 1979; Ray & Cremer, 1979; Pham Huu Chanh et al., 1984). Electroencephalogram (EEG) records showed generalized spike discharges prior to choreoathetosis (Ray & Cremer, 1979; Ray, 1980).

Mice presented far fewer symptoms than rats after oral dosing at comparable levels, diarrhoea being the only reportable observation (Glomot et al., 1980a).

Rats were injected intraperitoneally with $^{14}C$-labelled deltamethrin at the threshold doses required to produce the motor symptoms of toxicity of tremor and choreoathetosis. Blood and brain samples were analysed for their total radiolabel content, and were also extracted with ethyl acetate to determine the levels of extractable parent deltamethrin and 3-phenoxybenzyl-derived acid and the residual radiolabel after this extraction. There was a clear correlation between onset of symptoms and blood and brain levels of deltamethrin. It was found that certain threshold levels of parent deltamethrin in the blood and brain were required for symptoms development, and that the symptoms persisted for as long as this threshold was maintained (Rickard & Brodie, 1985).

Table 10. Acute toxicity of technical grade deltamethrin

| Species | Sex | Route | Vehicle | $LD_{50}$ (mg/kg body weight) | Reference |
|---|---|---|---|---|---|
| Rat | male | oral | sesame oil | 128 | Glomot & Chevalier (1976a) |
| | female | | | 139 | |
| | male | | PEG 200 | 67 | |
| | female | | | 86 | |
| Rat | male adult | | peanut oil | 52 | Kavlock et al. (1979) |
| | female adult | | | 31 | |
| | female weanling | | | 50 | |
| Rat | male adult | | peanut oil | 53 | Gaines & Linder (1986) |
| | female adult | | | 30 | |
| | female weanling | | | 48 | |
| Rat | male + female | | aqueous suspension with carboxy-methylcellulose | > 5000 (no mortality) | Audegond et al. (1981) |
| Rat | | dermal | – | 700 | Panshina & Sasinovich (1983) |
| Rat | male<br>female | | methylcellulose (1%) | > 2940 | Kynoch et al. (1979) |
| Rat | female adult | | xylene | > 800 | Kavlock et al. (1979) |
| Rat | male + female | inhalation (6 h) | dust | 600 $mg/m^3$ | Coombs & Clark (1978) |

Table 10 (*continued*)

| Species | Sex | Route | Vehicle | $LD_{50}$ (mg/kg body weight) | Reference |
|---|---|---|---|---|---|
| Rat | male adult | (2 h) | DMSO 10% aerosol | 940 mg/m$^3$ | Kavlock et al. (1979) |
| | female adult | | | > 785 mg/m$^3$ | |
| Rat | male + female | (1 h) | micronized powder | > 4620 mg/m$^3$ | Jackson & Hardy (1986) |
| Rat | | intraperitoneal | – | 58.8 | Panshina & Sasinovich (1983) |
| Rat | male | intraperitoneal | sesame oil | 209 | Glomot & Chevalier (1976b) |
| | female | | | 186 | |
| | male | | PEG 200 | 24 | Glomot & Chevalier (1976b) |
| | female | | | 25 | |
| Rat | male | intravenous | PEG 200 | 3.3 | Glomot & Chevalier, (1976c) |
| | female | | | 3.3 | |
| Rat | female adult | | acetone | 4 | Kavlock et al. (1979) |
| | female weanling | | | 1..8 | |
| Mouse | male | oral | sesame oil | 33 | Glomot & Chevalier (1976a) |
| | female | | | 34 | |
| | male | | PEG 200 | 21 | Glomot & Chevalier (1976a) |
| | female | | | 19 | |
| Mouse | | intraperitoneal | – | 33 | Panshina & Sasinovich (1983) |
| Mouse | male | intraperitoneal | sesame oil | 171 | Glomot & Chevalier (1976b) |
| | female | | | 166 | |

Table 10 (*continued*)

| | | | | | |
|---|---|---|---|---|---|
| Mouse | male<br>female | | PEG 200 | 18<br>12 | Glomot & Chevalier (1976b) |
| Mouse | male<br>female | | PEG 200 | 4.1<br>4.0 | Glomot & Chevalier (1976c) |
| Mouse | male<br>female | | glycerol formal | 5<br>5.8 | Glomot & Chevalier (1976c) |
| Dog | male + female | oral | in capsules | > 300<br>no<br>mortality | Glomot et al. (1977) |
| Dog | male + female | | PEG 200 | 2 | Glomot & Chevalier (1976c) |
| Rabbit | male<br>female | dermal | PEG 400 | > 2000<br>> 2000 | Clair (1977) |

Table 11 Acute Toxicity of some formulations

| Species | Sex | Route | Formulation | $LD_{50}$ (mg/kg body weight) | Reference |
|---|---|---|---|---|---|
| Rat | male, female | oral | 2.5% flowable formulation | 22 000 | Glomot et al. (1979) |
| Rat | male, female | oral | 2.5% wettable powder | > 15 000 | Glomot (1979) |
| Mouse | male, female | oral | 2.5% wettable powder | > 15 000 | Glomot et al. (1980a) |
| Dog | male, female | oral | 2.5% wettable powder | > 10 000 | Glomot et al. (1980b) |
| Rat | male, female | oral | 2.5% emulsifiable concentrate | 535 | Coquet (1977) |
| Rat | male, female | oral | 10 g/litre ULV | > 6 470 | Coquet (1977) |
| Rat | male, female | inhalation (4 h) | aerosol – 2.5% wettable powder | > 2 800 $mg/m^3$ | Clark et al. (1980) |

### 7.1.1 Mouse

Mice intravenously injected with deltamethrin showed intense tremors, convulsions, and ataxia, immediately after administration. Tachycardia and respiratory defects were also observed at higher dosages. Surviving animals appeared normal after 4–5 h. Immediately after intraperitoneal injection, jumping movements, slight convulsions and prostration, ptosis, tail hypertonicity, and cyanosis were observed. These toxic signs disappeared after 72 h in surviving animals.

Animals administered deltamethrin by gavage showed muscular stiffening and convulsions, 1 h after dosing. After 24 h, hypermotility, stereotype movements of the head, tachycardia, hypertonicity of the tail, and a few convulsions were observed. Behaviour and appearance were normal again after 48 h (Glomot & Chevalier, 1976a,c).

### 7.1.2 Rat

Rats intravenously injected with deltamethrin showed muscular contractions, piloerection, respiratory defects, convulsions, and paresis of the hind quarters, immediately following treatment. Surviving animals showed normal behaviour after 48 h. Immediately after intraperitoneal injection, tremor, convulsions, prostration, and cyanosis were observed. These toxic signs disappeared after 48 h in surviving animals. Animals administered deltamethrin by gavage showed motor incoordination, convulsions, respiratory defects, and hypomotility, shortly after dosing. Normal behaviour was observed after 3 days (Glomot & Chevalier, 1976c).

In an inhalation study (whole body exposure for 6 h), hyperactivity, grooming, and irritation were observed during exposure. The animals were hypersensitive to touch and noise and showed uncoordinated movements. Gross pathological investigation showed a gas-filled stomach and small intestine, and massive haemorrhage and degeneration in the lung (Coombs & Clark, 1978).

Rats were exposed (whole body exposure) for 4 h to an aerosol concentration of deltamethrin equal to 2.8 g/m$^3$, the highest attainable airborne concentration of a 2.5% wettable powder formulation. Approximately 80% of the total aerosol had a mean aerodynamic diameter of less than 5.5 µm. Dyspnoea and gasping were observed in exposed rats. Relative lung weights and macroscopic pathology were normal. There was no mortality (Clark et al., 1980).

### 7.1.3 *Rabbit*

Rabbits (10 males and 10 females) were treated with 2 g deltamethrin in 2 ml PEG 400 per kg body weight on 80 cm$^2$ of occluded shaved skin for 24 h. The animals were observed for 14 days. Two animals showed obvious erythema. No body weight changes or abnormal behaviour were observed. On histological observation of the liver, kidneys, and skin, small changes were observed, but these were common for this strain of rabbit and not related to treatment (Clair, 1977).

### 7.1.4 *Dog*

Dogs given oral doses of 100 mg deltamethrin/kg body weight or more showed transient hyperexcitability, akinesia, vomiting, and stiffness of the hind legs (Glomot et al., 1977).

Dogs orally dosed with 10.0 mg deltamethrin/kg body weight did not display any clinical signs related to treatment (Glomot et al., 1980b).

## 7.2 Irritation and sensitization

### 7.2.1 *Skin irritation*

Male albino rabbits (12 per group) weighing 2.5–3.5 kg were administered 0.5 g deltamethrin on either shaved intact or abraded skin. The occlusive patch was fixed on the skin for 23 h. Technical deltamethrin (98% purity) did not produce any irritant effects (Coquet, 1976a).

Male albino rabbits (6) weighing 2.5–2.9 kg were administered 0.5 ml of formulated deltamethrin (25 g/litre flowable suspension concentrate) to both shaved intact and abraded skin. The Primary Irritation Index after 24 h exposure of occluded sites was 1.2, i.e., slightly irritating (Glomot et al., 1981b).

An evaluation similar to the one described above was carried out for a 2.5% wettable powder concentrate deltamethrin formulation. Rabbits had a Primary Irritation Index of 2.41, i.e., moderately irritating. Moderate erythema continued for 72 h, while the oedema generally diminished, with the exception of scarified skin sites (Glomot et al., 1981c).

The skin irritation potentials of Decis emulsifiable concentrate 2.5% and Decis Flowable 2.5% were studied on rabbits and guinea-pigs with 0.05, 0.10, 0.5, 1, and 2.5% deltamethrin. The threshold irritative levels were 0.05 % for Decis emulsifiable concentrate and 2.5% for Decis Flowable. The intensity of irritation depended on the relative content of organic solvents and emulsifiers in the trade products. The water-soluble concentrate of Decis 2.5% caused negligible risk of contact irritative dermatitis (Bainova & Kaloyanova, 1985).

### 7.2.2 Eye irritation

Deltamethrin (0.1 g/animal) was administered into the conjunctival sac of the eyes of 6 male albino rabbits, weighing 2.5 kg, with or without rinsing 60 seconds after instillation. Deltamethrin produced transient irritating effects, both with and without rinsing (Coquet, 1976b).

Male albino rats (9) weighing between 2 and 3 kg were administered 0.1 ml of formulated deltamethrin (25 g/litre flowable suspension concentrate) in the conjunctival sac. Six of the treated eyes remained unwashed, while the remaining three were rinsed with lukewarm water 20–30 seconds after instillation. There was only transient clouding of the cornea in 2 animals 1 h after dosing (1 washed, 1 unwashed), which cleared by day 2. Low grade conjunctival irritation was noted among all animals initially, which disappeared following day 2 of observations (Glomot et al., 1981d).

A 2.5% deltamethrin formulation diluted 1/10 in distilled water (0.1 ml per rabbit) elicited a similar pattern of initial transient corneal clouding in 3 out of 9 rabbits examined, which cleared by day 4. The undiluted formulation (100 mg) administered in the conjunctival sac of rabbits produced increased involvement of the conjunctiva, iris, and cornea in all animals, generally moderate in severity, with low grade corneal opacity persisting in 2 rabbits until day 7 (1 washed, 1 unwashed) (Glomot et al., 1981e).

### 7.2.3 *Sensitization*

Deltamethrin (0.5 g/animal) was applied topically to the skin of albino guinea-pigs (10 male and female) 3 times per week, with a 2-day interval for 3 weeks, and once at the start of the fourth week. The preparation was covered with an occlusive patch for 48 h. On days 1 and 10, the guinea-pigs received an intradermal injection of 0.1 ml of Freund's adjuvant. The animals were challenged 12 days after the last application with 0.5 g deltamethrin. No sensitization was found (Guillot & Guilaine, 1977).

## 7.3 Short-term exposure

### 7.3.1 *Rat*

Male and female weanling Sprague-Dawley rats (20 of each sex per group) were dosed (by gavage) with 0, 0.1, 1, 2.5, or 10 mg deltamethrin in PEG 200/kg body weight per day for 13 weeks. No treatment-related effects were observed on food and water consumption, mortality, urinalysis, and haematology. Neurological examinations and ophthalmoscopy did not reveal any abnormalities. At the highest dose level, a slight hyperexcitibility was observed among some rats in week 6. Lower body weight gain was noted in males at 2.5 and 10 mg/kg. No clear treatment-related effects were noted in the results of laboratory investigations or on the weights of the organs. Gross and microscopic examination of a variety of tissues and organs did not show any treatment-related findings. Following the 13-week dosage period, 5 males and 5 females per group were allowed to recover for 4 weeks. No evidence of hyperexcitability was observed among the rats; body weight gain was slightly higher in the treated groups than in the controls. The no-observed-effect level was 1 mg/kg body weight (Hunter et al., 1977).

Four groups of CD rats (8 of each sex per group) were exposed to aerosolized deltamethrin (technical grade powder) for 6 h per day, 5 days a week, for 2 weeks, and for 4 days during a third week. Mean aerosol concentrations were 3, 9.6, and 56.3 mg a.i./$m^3$ with about 87% of respirable particles (diameter lower than 5.5 μm). No rats died as a result of exposure. Signs of irritation (agitated grooming and ptyalism) due to the powder were noted in all groups during exposure, with more pronounced toxic signs (ataxia and walking with arched backs) in the group receiving the highest dose tested. Male rats also showed a reduced body weight (–5%) in all groups. An elevation of the serum sodium ion content was noted at the two highest doses. No increased incidence of any particular lesion was observed in the high-dose group compared with the control group. Irritation and weight loss were only slight at 3 mg/$m^3$ and this can be considered as a no-effect level (Coombs et al., 1978).

### 7.3.2 Dog

Male and female beagle dogs (3–5/sex per group), 25 weeks of age, received a daily oral dose of 0, 0.1, 1, 2.5, or 10 mg deltamethrin/kg body weight in PEG 200 in gelatin capsules over 13 weeks. All treated groups showed reduced body weight gain, but this was not dose-related. Liquid faeçes were associated with all groups of treated dogs throughout the dosing period. Dilatation of the pupils was seen in dogs receiving 2.5 and 10 mg/kg per day. The sign was first seen 4–7 h after dosing and persisted throughout the day. The incidence of vomiting increased dose-dependently in all treated groups, except the group receiving 0.1 mg/kg. In the highest dose group, unsteadiness, body tremors, and jerking movements were seen, particularly in males, in weeks 2, 3, and 4. Excessive salivation was seen initially and diminished during the dosing period. After 5 and 12 weeks, depression of the gag reflex was noted in a proportion of animals in all treated groups. However, this was not considered to be of toxicological significance. Exaggeration or depression of the patellar reflex was observed in some animals in all treated groups after 5 and 12 weeks, mainly at 1, 2.5, or 10 mg/kg per day. Some animals in all treated groups showed depression of the flexor reflex. Dose levels of 2.5 and 10 mg deltamethrin/kg per day caused modification of the EEG pattern in some animals, 12 weeks following administration. Histopathological evaluations of tissues and organs, including the nervous system and muscle tissue, did not reveal any abnormalities that could be related to the administration of the compound. During recovery, the gag reflex continued to be depressed, whereas exaggeration of the patellar reflex was still seen in some dogs that had previously received 1 mg/kg per day (Chesterman et al., 1977).

## 7.4 Long-term exposure and carcinogenicity

### 7.4.1 *Mouse and rat*

Male and female Charles River CD-1 mice (80 of each sex per group) were fed dietary levels of deltamethrin of 0, 1, 5, 25, or 100 mg/kg, daily, for 24 months. There were no clear effects related to the administration of deltamethrin on general behaviour, mortality, body weight, and food consumption. Blood chemistry, haematology, and urine analysis parameters were normal after 12, 18, and 24 months (at the times of interim and terminal sacrifice). Microscopic examination of tissues did not reveal any lesions indicative of a compound-related effect. The tumour incidence was unaffected by deltamethrin administration. The no-observed-effect level was 100 mg/kg diet (Goldenthal et al., 1980a).

Deltamethrin was administered, by gavage, to C57BL/6 mice at 4 dose levels (0, 1, 4, and 8 mg/kg body weight) and to BDVI rats at 3 dose levels (0, 3, and 6 mg/kg body weight) on 5 days a week for 104 weeks. After completion of the treatment, the animals were observed until 120 weeks of age, when all survivors were killed. The treatment had a slight effect on body growth and survival rates, especially in the groups of mice and rats treated with the highest dose. In C57BL/6 mice, various types of tumours were observed in all treated groups. An increased incidence of lymphomas was observed in mice receiving deltamethrin at levels of 1 and 4 mg/kg body weight, but not in the group treated with 8 mg/kg body weight. No significant difference in the incidences of lung adenomas, liver-cell tumours, or other tumours was observed in treated groups compared with controls. In BDVI rats, an increased incidence of pituitary, thyroid, and mammary tumours was noted; however, no clear dose-response relationship was shown (Cabral et al., 1986). The details of this study were not available for evaluation.

Male and female Charles River CD rats (90 of each sex per group) were fed with 0, 2, 20, or 50 mg deltamethrin/kg diet for 2 years. A second control group (60 of each sex) was also used. Interim sacrifices (10 of each sex per group excluding control group 2) were made after 6, 12, and 18 months. No changes in general behaviour and appearance were observed in relation to treatment. Survival rate was similar for control and treated rats (50–67%). Rats in the 50 mg/kg group gained slightly less weight than control rats, whereas the food consumption was essentially the same. Ophthalmoscopic findings were generally similar for control and treated rats. No haematological and biochemical parameters were changed in a biologically significant way in relation to treatment at any time, except for a decrease in SGPT (serum glutamic pyruvic transaminase) activity at 6 months in the mid- and high-dose groups. Organ weights were not affected. The macroscopic and microscopic findings were common for the species and the strain, except for a slightly increased incidence of axonal degeneration in sciatic, tibial, and/or plantar nerves in the 20 and 50 mg/kg groups at 18 months, but not at termination. Thus, this was not considered to be indicative of a compound-related effect. The incidence of benign testicular tumours (interstitial cell adenomas) at terminal sacrifice in this study was: control group 1, 0/37; control group 2, 4/35; low-dose group 1/38; mid-dose group 1/30; high-dose group 6/38. The incidence seen in the high-dose group was considered to be spontaneous, because it was not significantly higher than in the second control group or in historical control groups (Goldenthal et al., 1980b; Richter & Goldenthal, 1983).

### 7.4.2 Dog

Deltamethrin dissolved in maize oil was administered in the diet to 64 beagle dogs (8 of each sex per group) at levels of 0, 1, 10, and 40 mg/kg for 24 months. This corresponds to 0, 0.025, 0.25, and 1 mg/kg body weight, respectively. Individual body weights and food consumption values were determined weekly. Ophthalmoscopic, haematological, biochemical, and urinanalysis examinations were conducted during the pre-test period and at 6, 12, 18, and 24 months of the study. Neurological examinations were conducted at approximately 1 year and before termination. No signs of overt toxicity were observed in any of the dogs. Body weight and food consumption values were similar for control and treated dogs. No compound-related effects were observed during the ophthalmoscopic and physical examinations. Although there were some random statistically significant differences between the control and other dose groups in the haematological and biochemical tests, physiologically significant changes were not observed at any interval in the study. Two treated and two control animals died during the study. No compound-related gross or microscopic changes were observed in the surviving dogs that were sacrificed and necropsied. Inflammatory, degenerative, and proliferative changes described were spontaneous in nature, or related to the estrous phase of the menstrual cycle, and unrelated to compound administration. On the basis of this study, it has been concluded that the no-observed-effect level is 40 mg/kg diet (equivalent to 1 mg/kg body weight per day) (IRDC, 198O).

## 7.5 Mutagenicity

### 7.5.1 Microorganisms

DNA repair tests in *Escherichia coli* were conducted at dose levels of 1250, 2500, or 5000 μg deltamethrin/ml. Deltamethrin was dissolved in dimethyl sulfoxide (DMSO) and 0.1 ml of the solution was spread on a plate. Growth inhibition was compared between DNA repair deficient mutants (p3478 and CM611) and wild types (W3110 and WP2). Partial precipitation of deltamethrin from the solution occurred when it came into contact with the aqueous bacterial growth medium. Deltamethrin did not have any damaging effects on DNA (Peyre et al., 1980).

Deltamethrin was examined for its mutagenic potential in the Ames test with 5 strains of *Salmonella typhimurium* (TA 1535, TA 1537, TA 1538, TA 98, and TA100) at doses of 2, 10, 50, 200, 500, 1000, or 5000 μg/plate, with and without S-9 mix (metabolic enzyme system). It was dissolved in DMSO and precipitated out of solution at concentrations of 200 μg/plate or more. Deltamethrin did not have any effect on the mutation rate in any of the strains at any of the concentrations tested (Peyre et al., 1980).

A similar Ames test was carried out at 0.2, 2, 20, 200, or 400 μg deltamethrin/plate with microsome enzymes. The compounds did not influence the number of revertants of the 5 strains (same as above) of *S. typhimurium*. Again, deltamethrin was dissolved in DMSO and precipitated out of solution at 200 μg/plate or more (Fouillet, 1976).

Kavlock et al. (1979) found deltamethrin not to be mutagenic in 2 assays with *S. typhimurium* at doses of 0–1000 μg/plate in DMSO, with or without metabolic activation. They also obtained negative results with *E. coli* at 10–1000 μg/plate as well as with *Saccharomyces cerevisiae* at concentrations of 1–5%, in both cases with and without metabolic activation. Deltamethrin was found not to be mutagenic in *S. typhimurium* strains TA100 and TA98, in the presence or absence of a rat liver activation system, using the plate incorporation assay and fluctuation tests. The compound, dissolved in DMSO, precipitated out of solution at 600 μg/plate (Pluijmen et al., 1984).

### 7.5.2 Cultured cells

Deltamethrin, dissolved in a mixture of cremaphor oil and ethanol (1:1), was applied to a culture of Chinese hamster ovary cells (CHO) at levels of 0.04, 0.2, 1.0, or 5.0 mmol/litre, with or without metabolic activation, and examined for chromosomal aberrations and sister chromatid exchanges (SCE). Because of the cytotoxic effect of cremaphor oil when combined with S-9 mix or deltamethrin, no cells would grow in the control dish with activation, or in the 5 mmol/litre deltamethrin dishes, either with or without metabolic activation. A high incidence of chromosomal aberrations and SCEs was observed in the dishes containing 1 mmol deltamethrin/litre, with activation. However, the absence of control values (both with and without activation) because of a broken test tube, made the interpretation equivocal. A second study was conducted in which deltamethrin was dissolved in DMSO and applied to the cells at levels of 0.001, 0.01, 0.1, or 0.2 mmol/litre, with or without metabolic activation. In this study, deltamethrin did not produce any cytotoxic effects and did not induce either chromosomal aberrations or SCEs in CHO cells. However, no positive controls were tested and only single plates were prepared per dose level (Sobels et al., 1978).

Deltamethrin was found not to be mutagenic in V79 Chinese hamster cells, in the presence or absence of hepatocytes. It is not known which solvent was used (Pluijmen et al., 1984).

### 7.5.3 Mouse

An *in vivo* cytogenetic test was conducted on mice (3 males and 3 females per group). Mice were treated orally with deltamethrin in sesame oil for 2 consecutive days at 5 or 10 mg/kg body weight. The incidence of chromosomal aberrations in bone marrow cells or micronuclei in the polychromatic erythrocytes of treated groups was, however, comparable to that of the control groups. No positive controls were tested (Sobels et al., 1978).

Deltamethrin was applied orally, once, at 15 mg/kg body weight to Swiss mice. A time-related effect on the chromosomes in bone marrow cells was observed by killing 2 animals every 3 h during 24 h. The report stated that the incidences of chromated aberrations were low and that there were no consistent time-related trends in the distribution of the aberrations. However, the time-related trend of aberrations was not reported. Again, no positive controls were tested (Sobels et al., 1978).

A dominant-lethal assay with deltamethrin was performed. Groups of 9–13 male mice were dosed orally at 3 mg/kg body weight in sesame oil for 7 days or at a single dose of 6 or 15 mg/kg body weight in sesame oil, and mated with 6–18 non-treated females. There were no effects on the rates of pre- and postimplantation losses, while the positive control, triethylene triphosphoramide (10 mg/kg body weight), reduced pregnancies in the second and third weeks after treatment and increased embryonal losses (Vannier & Glomot, 1977).

Deltamethrin in olive oil was administered orally to female Swiss mice at single or repeated (5 times at daily intervals) doses of 1.36, 3.4, or 6.8 mg/kg per day. Bone marrow smears were prepared 6, 24, or 48 h after treatment. No mutagenic activity was observed with deltamethrin, whereas the positive control, cyclophosphamide, induced a positive response (Polàkovà & Vargovà, 1983).

In a micronucleus test, a single dose of deltamethrin in corn oil was administered orally at 16 mg/kg body weight to Swiss CD-1 mice (5 of each sex per group). No mutagenic activity was observed with deltamethrin, whereas the positive controls, triethylenemelaminc and dimethylbenzanthracene, both induced positive responses (Vannier & Fournex, 1983).

### 7.5.4 *Appraisal*

Deltamethrin is not mutagenic or clastogenic in a variety of *in vitro* and *in vivo* test systems.

## 7.6 Teratological and reproductive effects

### 7.6.1 *Teratology*

#### 7.6.1.1 Mouse

Deltamethrin was dissolved in corn oil and administered by gastric intubation at doses of 0, 3.0, 6.0, or 12.0 mg/kg body weight on days 7–16 of gestation to groups of CD-1 mice. Mice were sacrificed on day 18 of gestation. There was a dose-related ($P < 0.001$) reduction in maternal weight gain during pregnancy and high-dose females gained 58% less weight than the controls. There was no dose-related mortality but dams in the high- and mid-dose groups became convulsive after dosing. Treatment did not affect the number of implantation sites, fetal mortality, fetal weights, or the number of sternal and caudal ossification centres.

A significant ($P < 0.01$) dose-related increase in the occurrence of supernumerary ribs was observed. No other dose-related skeletal or visceral anomalies were observed (Kavlock et al., 1979).

Pregnant female Swiss CD-1 SPF mice (24 per group) were given deltamethrin dissolved in sesame oil by oral intubation at dose-levels of 0, 0.1, 1, or 10 mg/kg body weight per day on days 6–17 of pregnancy. The animals were necropsied on day 18 of pregnancy. The numbers of implantation sites, fetal losses, and viable fetuses were not affected by treatment. There was a dose-related decrease in mean fetal weight. Apart from delayed ossification at all dose levels, skeletal examination revealed no abnormalities. A teratogenic effect was not observed (Glomot & Vannier, 1977).

In a complementary teratology study, pregnant female Swiss CD-1 mice were given deltamethrin dissolved in sesame oil by oral intubation at 0, 0.1, 1, or 10 mg/kg body weight per day from day 6 to day 17 of gestation. Females were either sacrificed on day 18 of gestation or allowed to litter for subsequent examination of pups on days 1 or 21 of lactation. The compound caused a moderate and transient retardation of development of the fetus at the 1 and 10 mg/kg body weight dose rate, but these effects were not observed on days 1 or 21 post-partum. There were no teratogenic effects related to treatment (Vannier & Glomot, 1982).

#### *7.6.1.2 Rat*

Pregnant female Sprague-Dawley rats (24 per group) received 0, 0.1, 1, or 10 mg deltamethrin/kg body weight per day by oral intubation on days 6–18 of pregnancy. Apart from 12 females in the control and 10 mg/kg groups, which were allowed to deliver, the dams were sacrificed and examined on day 21. There were no effects on reproduction or on the teratogenic parameters examined, except for slightly delayed ossification at the highest dose level (Glomot & Vannier, 1977).

Deltamethrin was dissolved in corn oil and administered by gastric intubation at doses of 0, 1.25, 2.5, or 5.0 mg/kg body weight on days 7–20 of gestation. Rats were sacrificed on day 21 of gestation. There was a dose-related reduction ($P < 0.01$) in maternal weight gain during pregnancy, and dams in the high-dose group gained only 80% of the control value. Treatment did not affect the number of implantation sites, fetal mortality, fetal weight, or the number of sternal and caudal ossification centres (Kavlock et al., 1979).

#### 7.6.1.3 Rabbit

Groups of 15 pregnant New Zealand White rabbits received deltamethrin dissolved in sesame oil at levels of 0, 1, 4, or 16 mg/kg body weight per day during days 6–19 of pregnancy. Examination was carried out on day 28 of gestation. The mean fetal loss was not dose-related. The mean fetal weight in the highest-dose group was decreased. Some malformations (hydrocephaly, exencephaly, and thoracogastroschisis) were observed in 2 fetuses of animals at the highest dose level. In a supplementary study, pregnant rabbits were similarly dosed with 16 mg/kg body weight per day; one fetus with spina bifida and shortened tail was detected among 69 apparently normal fetuses. Malformations were within the normal limits of the strain used and were not considered to be related to the treatment, despite the occurrence at the highest dose level only (Glomot & Vannier, 1977, 1978).

### 7.6.2 Reproduction studies

Groups of 10 male and 20 female Charles River rats were fed deltamethrin in the diet at 0, 2, 20, or 50 mg/kg and mated to begin a 3-generation, 2-litter (first generation, 3 litter) standard reproduction study. Parental body weights and food consumption were recorded during the study. After weaning of the second litter, the surviving parent rats were sacrificed and necropsied. Five male and 5 female pups of the $F_{3b}$ generation were necropsied. No changes relevant to treatment were observed in general behaviour or survival of parent rats or pups. The body weight of $F_0$ males of the 50 mg/kg group was decreased from week 11 onwards. There were some slight decreases in mean food consumption of $F_1$ male parent rats in the 50 mg/kg group. The basic reproduction indices (fertility, gestation, lactation, viability, and litter size) were not affected by the treatment. However, the mean pup weight in some litters, especially in the 50 mg/kg group, was slightly decreased in comparison to the controls on day 21 of lactation. Gross external examination did not reveal any abnormalities. No gross or microscopic lesions of treatment-related significance or significant effects on the organ weights of the $F_{3b}$ generation were observed (Wrenn et al., 1980).

Deltamethrin was dissolved in corn oil and administered by gastric intubation at doses of 0, 2.5, or 5.0 mg/kg body weight to Sprague-Dawley rats from day 7 of gestation to day 15 of lactation. The dams were allowed to litter and rear their young: litters were reduced at birth to 4 males and 4 females per litter. The pups were weighed weekly and examined for the development of eye-opening, startle reflex, and air-righting. The litters were weaned on day 22 post-partum and the males discarded. Weekly weighing of the females continued and at 6 weeks of age they were tested in a circular open-field. There were no effects on parturition, litter size, or pup viability. Weights at birth were similar for all groups, but a dose-related depression in growth was observed during the pre-weaning period. This early diminution in pre-weaning weight appeared to have little effect on the morphological and behavioural parameters measured (Kavlock et al., 1979).

## 7.7 Neurotoxicity and behavioural effects

Adult hens (10 per group) were gavaged with a single dose of 0, 500, 1250, or 5000 mg deltamethrin/kg body weight suspended in corn oil or 0 or 100 mg/kg body weight dissolved in sesame oil. During 21 days, observations were made on mortality, health, neurotoxic signs, and body weight. Deltamethrin did not induce any clinical, macroscopic, or histological signs of delayed neurotoxicity (Ross et al., 1978).

Groups of 5 male and 5 female Wistar rats were administered 25 mg deltamethrin/kg body weight in 10 mg corn oil/kg on 2 consecutive days. Controls received 10 mg corn oil/kg body weight. A tilting plane test was performed every second day from day 4 to day 16 of the study. Two male rats died at 25 mg/kg. No effect was found on the slip-angle (Davies et al., 1983).

The effects of deltamethrin were studied in a rat performance test that arranged for milk delivery after every fortieth lever press. Deltamethrin (1–8 mg/kg body weight, given orally, 2 h before the test) produced both dose-related increases in pause duration and decreases in response rate. Deltamethrin was also studied using a conditional flavour-aversion test. Deltamethrin-treated, trained rats displayed an aversion to saccharin that was greatest at 2 mg/kg (Macphail, 1981).

The neurological effects of the 4 synthetic pyrethroids, resmethrin, permethrin, cypermethrin, and deltamethrin, have been investigated in the rat to establish whether there is a correlation between the clinical-functional status of the animal and peripheral nerve damage, as measured biochemically (Rose & Dewar, 1983). Neuromuscular dysfunction was assessed by means of the inclined plane test and peripheral nerve damage by reference to β-glucuronidase and β-galactosidase activity increases in nerve tissue homogenates from treated and control animals. A transient functional impairment was found in animals treated with any one of the 4 pyrethroids tested and in all cases this was greatest at the end of the 7-day dosing regimen (deltamethrin doses of 5–20 mg/kg per day in arachis oil). Significant increases in β-glucuronidase and β-galactosidase activities were found 3–4 weeks after the start of dosing, in the distal portion of the sciatic/posterior tibial nerves from permethrin-, cypermethrin-, and deltamethrin-treated animals, but no changes were found in resmethrin-treated animals. It is concluded, therefore, that there is no direct correlation between the time-course of the neuromuscular dysfunction and the neurobiochemical changes. This suggests that these pyrethroids have at least two distinct actions – a short-term pharmacological effect at near-lethal dose levels and a more long-term neurotoxic effect that results in sparse axonal nerve damage.

To better characterize the behavioural toxicity of pyrethroid insecticides, comparisons were made of the effects of cismethrin and deltamethrin exposure on motor activity and the acoustic startle response in male Long-Evans rats (Crofton & Reiter, 1984). Acute dose-effect, acute time-course, and 30-day repeated-exposure determinations of 1-h motor activity were made using figure-eight mazes. The acoustic startle response was measured to a 13-kHz, 120-dB(A), 40-millisecond tone at each of 3 background white noise levels (50, 65, and 80 dB). Deltamethrin (0, 2, 4, 6, or 8 mg/kg body weight) or cismethrin (0, 6, 12, 18, or 24 mg/kg) were administered orally in 0.2 ml/kg corn oil. Cismethrin and deltamethrin produced similar dose-dependent decreases in motor activity. The time course of onset and recovery for this decreased activity was rapid (1–4 h). No cumulative effects on motor activity of a 30-day exposure to 2 mg deltamethrin/kg per day or 6 mg cismethrin/kg per day were found. The effects of cismethrin and deltamethrin on the acoustic startle response were dissimilar: deltamethrin produced a dose-dependent decrease in amplitude and an increase in latency, and cismethrin produced an increase in amplitude and no change in latency. The differential effects of cismethrin (Type I pyrethroids) and deltamethrin (Type II pyrethroids) on the acoustic startle response may be related to the contrasting effects previously shown with neurophysiological and/or neurochemical techniques (see Appendix 1).

## 7.8 Miscellaneous effects

Analgesic effects of deltamethrin for thermic (hot plate test, 60 °C) and mechanical stimuli were investigated in mice and rats, respectively. Deltamethrin prolonged the response-time to these tests. Although this action was not significant at 500 mg deltamethrin/kg body weight given orally, the reaction time was increased at 1000 and 1500 mg/kg given orally in aqueous suspension with 10% gum arabic (Chanh et al., 1981).

In rats, treatment with deltamethrin increased mean arterial pressure and aortic output (Forshaw & Bradbury, 1983). The cardiovascular effects of deltamethrin were due to both increased catecholamine release in peripheral vascular beds, and to a direct positive inotropic effect on the heart.

Krasnjih & Pavlova (1985) demonstrated induction of microsomal oxygenases in rats 20 h after a single administration of 1/2 $LD_{50}$. Daily administration of 1/10th $LD_{50}$ for 2 months reduced acetylcholinesterase activity in the serum, erythrocytes, liver, and cerebrum. It also led to some changes in the aspartate aminotransferase activity and the urea and protein contents of serum.

When rats were dosed orally with a single dose of 1/2 $LD_{50}$ or 3 daily doses of 1/5 $LD_{50}$ deltamethrin, the activities of transferrin and ceruloplasmin in plasma, 20 h after dosing, were unchanged. After the single dose, microsomal mono-oxygenase activity was increased by 87%, and after the 3 doses, it was increased by 290% (Kagan et al., 1986).

## 7.9 Potentiation

Deltamethrin was hydrolysed *in vitro* by esterases in blood, brain, kidney, liver, and stomach preparations of mice. Pretreatment of mice with the oxidase inhibitor, piperonyl butoxide (PBO), or the esterase inhibitor, *S,S,S*-tributylphosphorotrithioate (DEF), delayed metabolism of intraperitoneally administered deltamethrin. PBO or DEF made mice more sensitive to deltamethrin (Ruzo et al., 1979).

Plasma esterases, in addition to hepatic esterases, play a role in the metabolism of deltamethrin in mammals and cause its rapid detoxification by the oral route. In a potentiation study, a range of esterase inhibitors, consisting mainly of organophosphorus insecticides, was given to male rats in oral doses that inhibited 50% of the plasma cholinesterase. After 15 min, or 2 or 24 h, an oral $LD_{50}$ dose of deltamethrin EC formulation was given, which showed potentiation with azinphos ethyl, omethoate, and dichlorvos. It appears that users must handle deltamethrin in these combinations very carefully because of their high toxicity. Acephate, monocrotophos, phosphamidon, parathion methyl, and the 2 controls did not act as potentiators (Audegond et al., 1988).

## 7.10 Mechanism of toxicity (mode of action)

Deltamethrin is classified as a Type II pyrethroid. For the mode of action of pyrethroids in general see Appendix 1.

The lowest concentration of deltamethrin to have an effect in crayfish stretch receptor neurones on sodium channels was

$10^{-12}$ mol/litre, but the response of the preparation to gamma-aminobutyric acid (GABA) appeared to be unaffected by concentrations of deltamethrin up to $10^{-7}$ mol/litre. Although $10^{-6}$ mol/litre deltamethrin had a slight effect on the GABA response of the dactyl abductor muscle, it appears that the majority of the effects of cyano-pyrethroids in invertebrates could be accounted for solely by their action on sodium channels (Chalmers et al., 1987).

Pyrethroid-induced motor symptoms, i.e., deltamethrin-induced writhing and cismethrin-induced tremor, were studied, using a number of pharmacological agents, in intact conscious rats and spinal rats. The results suggest that pyrethroid-induced motor symptoms, i.e., writhing and tremor, are mediated via a spinal site of action, probably involving interneurones. Deltamethrin-induced "non-motor" symptoms, i.e., increase in brain blood flow and blood glucose may result from a supraspinal component of deltamethrin activity. In contrast, the cardiovascular effects of deltamethrin are mediated via a peripheral site of action (Bradbury et al., 1983).

Tissue culture experiments have shown that the dorsal root ganglion is more sensitive to deltamethrin than the spinal cord or peripheral nerve fibres. The morphological alterations observed in the neuronal bodies of the ganglia may reflect some perturbation of the ionic equilibrium ($Na^+$ and $Ca^+$) (Souyri, 1985).

The results of several other, sometimes very detailed and specialized, studies on the mode of action of deltamethrin have been reported. Because these results do not basically influence the present evaluation of deltamethrin, they are not reviewed in detail. The interested reader is referred to the following publications and a review by Bidet et al. (1988): Aldridge et al. (1978), Duclohier & Georgescauld (1979), Gray et al. (1980), Jacques et al. (1980), Miller & Adams (1980), Gammon et al. (1981), Pichon (1981), Brodie & Aldridge (1982), Dyball (1982), Parkin & LeQuesne (1982), Ray (1982), Staatz et al. (1982), Brodie (1983), Takahashi & LeQuesne (1983), Berlin et al. (1984), Prasada Rao et al. (1984), Bloomquist & Soderlund (1985), Brodie (1985), Brodie & Opacka (1985), Bloomquist et al. (1986), Chinn & Narahashi (1986), Doherty et al. (1986),

Forshaw & Ray (1986), Staatz-Benson & Hosko (1986), Brooks & Clark (1987), Forshaw et al. (1987), Leibowitz et al. (1987), Lummis et al. (1987), Stein et al. (1987).

## 7.11 Experimental studies on antidotes

Treatments capable of counteracting acute deltamethrin poisoning have been investigated in experimental animals. Ray & Cremer (1979) have proposed atropine, Gammon et al. (1982), phenobarbital and diazepam, and Bradbury et al. (1981, 1983), mephenesin.

In order to find a therapeutically usable antagonist, pharmacological screening was carried out by Dumont (1978), Dumont & Chifflot (1978), and Dumont & Laurent (1979). The outcome was that barbiturates are therapeutically active, but that the most efficient product is ethyl carbamate. Cotonat et al. (1987) and Fournier (1988) have confirmed that ethyl carbamate is an effective treatment for severe deltamethrin poisoning. However, a serious drawback is its antimitotic activity. Leclercq et al. (1986) began by evaluating the activity of common anticonvulsants, such as diazepam and clomethiazole. These products exhibited satisfactory activity in rats and dogs (Thiebault et al., 1985, 1988).

Phenoprobamate and mephenesin carbamate have been shown to be effective in the experimental treatment of deltamethrin poisoning (Cotonat et al. 1987; Leclercq et al. 1986). A summary of the results of the antidote studies can be found in Bleys et al. (1986). Clinical trials based on these studies will be undertaken (unpublished information given to the IPCS by Roussel-Uclaf).

The therapeutic effects of methocarbamol have also been shown by Hiromori et al. (1986). However, the mechanism underlying this activity is not clear as the actual anticonvulsant activity is weak.

It appears that for the time being barbiturates, and especially diazepam, offer the safest symptomatic treatment in case of deltamethrin poisoning. Advice on treatment for deltamethrin poisoning is given in the IPCS *Deltamethrin health and safety guide* (WHO, 1989).

# 8. EFFECTS ON MAN

## 8.1 General population – poisoning incidents

A few cases of attempted suicides with deltamethrin formulations (mainly EC), all non-fatal, have been reported in anti-poison centres. Two typical cases are described below.

The first poisoning case in a 13-year-old girl who ingested voluntarily 200 ml of a 2.5% EC formulation (5 grams of deltamethrin) was described by Rousselin (1983). After an unknown time, she lost consciousness and developed generalized muscle cramps, myosis, and tachycardia. Treatment in hospital was as follows: gastric lavage, PAM 0.5 mg; atropine 2 mg; sodium nitrite, 3% sodium thiosulfate; and, lastly, high doses of diazepam. She completely recovered in 48 h.

A second poisoning case, concerning another attempted suicide by a 23-year-old man, was reported by Foulhoux (1988). After oral absorption of 70 cc of a 2.5% EC formulation (1.75 g pure deltamethrin), there were no neurological signs in this patient. Digestive and hepatic signs occurred, probably due to absorption of the solvent, since determination of xylene in plasma was positive. The patient was treated with haemodialysis, phenobarbital, lidocaine, and provoked alkaline diuresis. Recovery followed within 48 h.

## 8.2 Occupational exposure

### *8.2.1 Acute toxicity – poisoning incidents*

Rousselin (1983) described a case of poisoning in an agricultural worker as a result of skin contamination with a liquid containing 5 g deltamethrin/litre. He developed paraesthesia in the legs, mouth, and tongue, and diarrhoea. Following washing of the skin and administration of antihistamines, he still had tingling sensations in his toes after 24 h, but was fully recovered after 48 h.

Outbreaks of acute deltamethrin and fenvalerate poisoning occurred in cotton growers in China in 1982–84. The farmers handled the pyrethroid insecticides without taking any precautions. Skin sensations occurred in more than 90% of the exposed workers. After repeated spraying in the cotton fields, the mild cases presented severe headaches, dizziness, fatigue, nausea, and anorexia, with transient changes in the EEG. A severe case developed muscular fasciculation, repetitive discharges in the EMG, and frequent convulsions, which were treated with diazepam and phenobarbital. However, in follow-up studies, all workers were found to have made complete recovery, and the prognosis of acute pyrethroid poisoning was found to be good (He, 1987; Tong Ying, 1988).

More recently He et al. (1989) reviewed 573 cases of acute pyrethroid poisoning reported in the Chinese medical literature during 1983–88. Among these there were 325 cases of acute deltamethrin poisoning: 158 occupational, due to inappropriate handling, and 167 accidental, mostly due to ingestion. Two patients died of convulsions. All others recovered with symptomatic and supportive treatment within 1–6 days. Clinical manifestations are well reviewed (He, 1987).

### 8.2.2 Effects of short- and long-term exposure

Among plant workers dermally exposed to technical deltamethrin or its formulations, cutaneous and mucuous manifestations were observed. Initial lesions were tenacious and painful pruritus, especially observed after exposure to hot water or perspiration, followed by a blotchy local burning sensation with blotchy erythema for about 2 days. Thereafter, slight and regular desquamation, restricted to the contaminated area, occurred. Cutaneous signs were sometimes accompanied by itching of the face (mainly around the mouth) and/or rhinorrhoea or lachrymation (Husson, 1978).

Apart from the above-mentioned effects, no long-term or persistent effect, or allergic diseases were reported in 70 workers, who had been exposed from 1977–87 in a deltamethrin-manufacturing and -formulating plant in France (unpublished Roussel Uclaf information supplied to the IPCS, 1988).

A field study was carried out in the United Kingdom with three unprotected operators and one operator wearing hood, gloves, and respirator, all of whom were involved in orchard spraying with deltamethrin according to normal field practice. The exposure time was 3.5 h. No changes were found in blood cell counts, total protein, urea, alkaline phosphates, $\gamma$-GT and SGOT in blood. Little deltamethrin was found in the respirator pad and no residues were found in the urine. There was no decrease in nerve conduction velocity, but a slight tendency to the opposite reaction. None of the operators experienced facial sensations (Hewson & Burgess, 1981).

Four operators were evaluated by the same authors during normal field applications of deltamethrin lasting one day. Three of the operators did not wear any protection on their heads or hands, while one wore hood, gloves, and a respirator. Motor and sensory nerve conduction velocities were determined as well as haematological and biochemical parameters and urinalysis. No changes were observed in the blood parameters measured and no residues were found in the urine samples. Furthermore, nerve conduction velocity did not decrease. Residues were primarily confined to gloves and legs. None of the operators experienced facial sensations (Hewson & Burgess, 1981).

Persons exposed to deltamethrin for 7–8 years in production and formulation were subjected to clinical and haematological examinations. Evaluations were conducted at several plants. There were no measurable effects other than transient irritation of cutaneous and mucous membranes, which was without sequelae. Adequate precautionary measures, such as the wearing of gloves and face masks, provided protection from exposure (Foulhoux, 1981).

A medical survey of agricultural workers involved in the use and application of EC and WP formulations of deltamethrin in Yugoslavia revealed no untoward symptoms of exposure, other than itching and burning of the face, and nasal hypersecretion. Medical examinations included chest X-ray, ECG, liver function tests, neurological examinations (eye tonometry, Goldman perimetry, dark adaptation ability), kidney function tests, and whole blood and plasma cholinesterase activity. No adverse effects were noted. The need for the proper use of masks and gloves, as well as good personal hygiene (e.g., washing), was emphasized (Plestina, 1981).

Five healthy volunteers, 16–40 years of age, were exposed to deltamethrin during 5 days of spraying in a cotton field in India in 1981. A sixth volunteer was engaged in mixing and loading the emulsion during the same period. Spraymen were exposed for 7 h daily. No one complained about any symptoms. No clinical abnormalities were detected, particularly with respect to neurological examination (muscle power, coordination, tremors, reflexes, and both light and deep sensations). No cardiovascular, respiratory, or abdominal abnormalities were detected, and no skin, mucous membrane, or eye lesions were observed during, and after cessation of, exposure (Trivedi, 1981).

A health survey was carried out among spraymen exposed to 2.5% deltamethrin emulsifiable concentrate in cotton fields in China. The subjects were exposed to deltamethrin at concentrations of 0.022–24.070 $\mu g/m^3$ in the air of the respiratory zone and 0.013–0.347 $\mu g/cm^2$ of skin contact. One half of the 44 sprayers complained of itching and burning sensations on their faces. A few miliary red papules also appeared on the face of one of them, but no signs of acute deltamethrin poisoning were noticed during physical examination. There were no significant differences in the sodium, potassium, and urea contents of the serum, the sodium, potassium, ATPase, and serotonin contents of whole blood, and the levels of 3-methyl-4-hydroxymandelic acid and 5-hydroxy-indoleacetic acid in the urine between the subjects examined and the controls. Deltamethrin in the urine of spraymen was below the detection limit of 0.10 μg/litre (Wang et al., 1988).

Mestres et al. (1985) measured the dermal and inhalation exposure of mixer/applicators who applied deltamethrin to vegetable crops in greenhouses in southern France and of workers who picked fruit from treated trees in the same area. This appeared to be less than 0.0065% of the toxic dose per hour with a mask and 0.0017%, without a mask.

In a department producing an aerosol of the domestic Bulgarian insecticide "Dekazol" containing 0.02, 0.04, or 0.08% deltamethrin, severe subjective complaints of sensory irritation were found because of the high levels of contamination of the workplace air with deltamethrin and also dermal contamination. Skin irritation with conjunctivitis and irritation of the respiratory system were discovered in all 25 workers. Two of them had contact urticaria. Patch testing with 0.03% deltamethrin showed a positive reaction in 5 out of 23 workers tested (Bainova et al., 1986).

## 8.3 Clinical studies

Three formulations of deltamethrin in petroleum solvent were patch tested on 37 human volunteers (double blind trial against solvent control). A dose of 20 μl of a 1% suspension in water, of a 25 g/litre emulsifiable concentrate was put on the facial skin of each volunteer, with a randomized distribution of control and active dilution. The duration of the irritation was short (from some minutes to 1 h) and the severity was described as slight by most of the volunteers. No skin damage was reported (Foulhoux et al., 1981).

# 9. PREVIOUS EVALUATIONS BY INTERNATIONAL BODIES

The Joint FAO/WHO Meeting on Pesticide Residues (JMPR) discussed and evaluated deltamethrin at its meetings in 1980, 1981, 1982, 1984, 1985, 1986, 1987, and 1988 (FAO/WHO, 1981, 1982, 1983, 1985a, 1986a, 1986b, 1988a,b,c). In 1982, an acceptable daily intake (ADI) of 0–0.01 mg/kg body weight was established.

The following Maximum Residue Limits (MRLs), in mg/kg, resulted from these evaluations:

| | |
|---|---|
| tea | 10.0 |
| hops dry, wheat bran unprocessed[a] | 5.0 |
| coffee beans (post-harvest) | 2.0 |
| wheat wholemeal,[a] cereal grains,[a] (ph) lentil (dry),[a] beans (dry),[a] field pea (dry)[a] | 1.0 |
| straw and fodder (dry) of cereal grains, legume animal feeds (dry weight), leafy vegetables | 0.5 |
| brassica leafy vegetables,[a] edible peel of fruiting vegetables[a] | 0.2 |
| bulb vegetables, edible peel of assorted fruits, legume vegetables, oilseeds, pome fruits, wheat flour[a] | 0.1 |
| artichokes, bananas, clementines, coco beans, grapes, kiwi fruit, oranges (sweet, sour), stone fruits/strawberries | 0.05 |

[a] Not yet confirmed by Codex Alimentarius Commission (FAO/WHO, 1986c, and 1988c).

| | |
|---|---|
| legume oilseeds, melons, mushrooms, pineapples, root and tuber vegetables, milks[a] | 0.01 |

WHO has classified deltamethrin as a moderately hazardous technical product in normal use (WHO, 1988). A Data Sheet on deltamethrin (No. 50) has been issued (WHO/FAO, 1984).

[a] Not yet confirmed by Codex Alimentarius Commission (FAO/WHO, 1986c, and 1988c).

# REFERENCES


ADENEY, R.J., GRZYWACZ, D., & MATTHIESSEN P. (1980) The acute toxicities of pyrethrin analogues to *Sarotherodon mossambicus* (Peters), Centre for Overseas Pest Research, 6 pp. (Unpublished proprietary data submitted to WHO by Roussel Uclaf).

AKHTAR, M.H. (1984) Metabolism of deltamethrin by cow and chicken liver enzyme preparations. J. agric. food Chem., **32:** 258-262.

AKHTAR, M.H., HAMILTON, R.M.G., & TRENHOLM, H.L. (1985) Metabolism, distribution and excretion of deltamethrin by leghorn hens. J. agric. food Chem., **33**: 610-617.

AKHTAR, M.H., MARTIN, K.E., & TRENHOLM, H.L. (1986) Fate of $^{14}$C-deltamethrin in lactating dairy cows. J. agric. food Chem., **34:** 753-758.

AKHTAR, M.H., DANIS, C., TRENHOLM, H.L.., & MARTIN, K.E. (1987) Residues in milk and tissues of lactating dairy cows fed deltamethrin for 28 consecutive days. J. agric. food Chem.,

ALDRIDGE, W.N., CLOTHIER, B., FORSHAW, P., & JOHNSON, M.K., PARKER, V.H., PRICE, R.J., SKILLETER, D.N., VERSCHOYLE, R.D., STEVENS, C. (1978) The effect of DDT and the pyrethroids cismethrin and decamethrin on the acetyl choline and cyclic nucleotide content of rat brain. Biochem. Pharmacol., **27:** 1703-1706.

ALINIAZEE, M.T. & CRANHAM, J.E. (1980) Effects of four synthetic pyrethroids on a predatory mite, *Typhlodroums pyri,* and its prey, *Panonychus ulmi,* on apples in southeast England. Environ. Entomol., **9:** 436-439.

ARZONE, A. & VIDANO, C. (1978) [Azione sull'ape di etiofencaus, decamethrin e ciexatin.] Apic. mod., **69:** 157-162, (in Italian)..

ATKINS, E.L., KELLUM D., & NEUMAN, K.J. (1976) Effect of pesticides on apiculture project No. 1449: The annual report, University of California Riverside, pp. 536-567. .

AUDEGOND, L., CATEZ, D., FOULHOUX, P., FOURNEX, R., LE RUMEUR, C., L'HOTELLIER, M., & STEPNIEWSKI, J.P. (1988) Potentialisation de la toxicité de la deltaméthrine par les insecticides organophosphorés (Unpublished proprietary data submitted to WHO by Roussel Uclaf).

AUDEGOND L., COLLAS E., & GLOMOT R. (1981) RU 22974 (deltamethrin) single administration study by oral route in the rat (the compound is given as a suspension) (Unpublished report RU-81239/A, submitted to WHO by Roussel Uclaf).

BAINOVA, A. & KALOYANOVA, F. (1985) [Study of allergenic and irritating effect of synthetic pyrethroids on skin.] Hig. Zdrav., **28**(2): 19-21 (in Bulgarian).

BAINOVA, A., MIHAVSKI, M., ISMIROVA, N., & BENCHEV, V. (1986) Specific skin irritation after contact with specific pyrethroids. 6th Congress of Bulgarian Dermatologists, Varna, 2-5 October, 1986, (Abstract No. 74) (in Bulgarian).

BAKER, P.G. & BOTTOMLEY, P. (1982) Determination of residues of synthetic pyrethroids in fruit and vegetables by gas-liquid and high-performance liquid chromatography. Analyst, **107**: 206-212.

BALDRY, D.A.T., EVERTS, J., ROMAN, B., BOON VON OCHSSEE, G.A., & LAVEISSIERE, C. (1981) The experimental application of insecticides from a helicopter for the control of riverine populations of *Glossina tachinoides* in West Africa. Part VIII: The effects of two spray applications of OMS-570 (endosulfan) and of OMS 1998 (decamethrin) on G. *tachinoides* and non-target organisms in Upper Volta. Trop. Pest Manage., **27**(1): 83-110.

BEAVERS, J.B. & FINK, R. (1977a) Actue oral $LD_{50}$ Mallard duck technical DECIS final report, (Unpublished report WI77.06.06/A, submitted to WHO by Roussel Uclaf). Wildlife International.

BERLIN, J.R., AKERA, T., BRODY, T.M., & MATSUMURA, F. (1984) The inotropic effects of a synthetic pyrethroid decamethrin on isolated guinea pig atrial muscle. Eur. J. Pharmacol., **98**: 313-322.

BIDET, D., DUMONT, C., FOULHOUX, P., FOURNEX, R., & ROUGERON, C. (1988) Mechanisms responsible for the toxicity of deltamethrin and other pyrethroids. (Unpublished document, submitted to WHO by Roussel Uclaf).

BLEYS, M., COTONAT, J., FOULHOUX, P. (1986) Lettre a l'éditeur, J. Toxicol. clin. exp., **6**(3): 211-212.

BLOOMQUIST, J.R., SODERLUND, D.M. (1985) Neurotoxic insecticides inhibit GABA-dependent chloride uptake by mouse brain vesicles. Biochem. biophys. Res. Commun., **133**(1): 37-43.

BLOOMQUIST, J.R., ADAMS, P.M., & SODERLUND, D.M. (1986) Inhibition of gamma-aminobutyric acid-stimulated chloride flux in mouse brain vesicles by polychlorocycloalkane and pyrethroid insecticides. Neurotoxicology, **7**(3): 11-20.

BOCQUET, J.C., PASTRE, P., ROA, L., & BAUMEISTER, R. (1980) Etude de l'action de la deltaméthrine sur *Apis mellifera* en conditions de plein-champ. Phytiatr. Phytopharm., **29**: 83-92.

BOCQUET, J.C., PASTRE, P., & BAUMEISTER, R. (1983) Bilan de cinq années d'études de l'effet de la deltaméthrine sur abeilles en conditions naturelles. 6ème Congrès International du Colza, Paris, mai 1983.

BOUCHE, M.B. & FAYOLLE, L. (1979) Tests carried out with Procida compound Decis EC 2.5 on earthworms lethal effect in relation with time (Unpublished proprietary report No. INRA-VT-79.05.22/78.10.10/A, submitted to WHO by Roussel Uclaf).

BOWMAN, H. & CARPENTER, M. (1987) Determination of photodegradation of $^{14}$C-deltamethrin in aqueous solution (Unpublished proprietary report ABC LABS 35491, submitted to WHO by Roussel Uclaf).

BRADBURY, J.E., GRAY, A.J., & FORSHAW, P. (1981) Protection against pyrethroid toxicity in rats with mephenesin. Toxicol. appl. Pharmacol., **60**: 382.

BRADBURY, J.E., FORSHAW, P.J., GRAY, A.J., & RAY, D.E. (1983) The action of mephenesin and other agents on the effects produced by two neurotoxic pyrethroids in the intact and spinal rat. Neuropharmacology, **22**(7): 907-914.

BRODIE, M.E. (1983) Correlations between cerebellar cyclic GMP and motor effects induced by deltamethrin: independence of olivo-cerebellar tract. Neurotoxicology, **4**(4): 1-11.

BRODIE, M.E. (1985) Deltamethrin infusion into different sites in the neuraxis of freely moving rats. Neurobehav. Toxicol. Teratol., **7**(1): 51-55.

BRODIE, M.E. & ALDRIDGE, W.N. (1982) Elevated cerebellar cyclic GMP levels during the deltamethrin-induced motor syndrome. Neurobehav. Toxicol. Teratol., **4**: 109-113.

BRODIE, M.E. & OPACKA, J. (1985) Dissociation between circling behaviour and striatal dopamine activity following unilateral deltamethrin administration to rats. Naunyn-Schmiedeberg's Arch. Pharmacol., **331**: 341-346.

BROOKS, M.W. & CLARK, J.M. (1987) Enhancement of norepinephrine release from rat brain synaptosomes by alpha cyano pyrethroids. Pestic. Biochem. Physiol., **28**: 127-139.

BUCCAFUSCO, R.J., ELLS, S.J., & CARY, G.A. (1977a) Acute toxicity of NRDC 161 to bluegill (*Lepomis macrochirus*) under dynamic test conditions, E.G. & G. Bionomics Aquatic Toxicology Laboratory, 12 pp. (Unpublished proprietary data submitted to WHO by Roussel Uclaf).

BUCCAFUSCO R.J., ELLS, S.J., & CARY, G.A. (1977b) Acute toxicity of NRDC 161 (Decamethrine) to Channel Catfish (*Ictalurus punctatus*), E.G. & G. Bionomics Aquatic Toxicology Laboratory, 7 pp. (Unpublished proprietary data supplied to WHO by Roussel Uclaf).

CABRAL, J.R.P., GALENDO, D., LAVAL, M., & LYANDRUT, N. (1986) Carcinogenicity study of the pesticide deltamethrin in mice and rats. Summary Report in Poster Session at IUPAC Meeting, Ottawa, August 1986.

CARY, G.A. (1978) Kinetics of 14C-NRDC-161 in a model aquatic ecosystem, E.G. & G. Bionomics Aquatic Toxicology Laboratory. (Unpublished proprietary report BW-78-2-075, submitted to WHO by Roussel Uclaf).

CHALMERS, A.E., MILLER, T.A, & OLSEN, R.W. (1987) Deltamethrin: a neurophysiological study of the sites of action. Pestic. Biochem. Physiol., **27**: 36-41.

CHAMBON, A. & LEPAILLEUR, H. (1984) Etude de l'effet toxique de la deltaméthrine (produit technique > 98%) et de la formulation CE 25 g/l Decis vis-à-vis de l'espèce de vers (*Eisenia fetida andrei*) (Unpublished proprietary report IRCHA-84.30.07/F, submitted to WHO by Roussel Uclaf).

CHANH, P.H., NAVARRO-DELMASURE, C., CHANH, A.P.H., LEAN, C.S., ZIADE, F., & SAMAHA, F. (1981) Analgesic effects of decamethrin, Surg. Transplant., **9**: 503-504.

CHAPMAN, R.A. & HARRIS, C.R. (1981) Persistence of four pyrethroid insecticides in a mineral and organic soil. J. environ. Sci. Health, **B16**: 605-615.

CHAPMAN, R.A., TU, C.M., HARRIS, C.R., & COLE, C. (1981) Persistence of five pyrethroid insecticides in sterile and natural, mineral and organic soil. Bull. Environ. Contam. Toxicol, **26**: 513-519.

CHESTERMAN, H., HEYWOOD, R., PERKIN, C.J., BEARD, D., STREET, E., & PRENTICE, D.E. (1977) RU 22974. Oral toxicity study in Beagle dogs, Huntingdon, Huntingdon Research Centre, (Unpublished report RSL 253/7751/A3, submitted to WHO by Roussel Uclaf).

CHINN, K. & NARAHASHI, T. (1986) Stabilization of sodium channel states by deltamethrin in mouse neuroblastoma cells. J. Physiol., **380**: 191-207.

CLAIR, M. (1977) RU 22974 DECIS. Acute toxicity in the rabbit by percutaneous administration. Joinville-le-Pont, Institut Français de Recherches et Essais Biologique (Unpublished report IFREB- R 770257.1/A, submitted to WHO by Roussel Uclaf).

CLARK, G.C., JACKSON, G.C., & ALEXANDER, D.J. (1980) Acute inhalation toxicity in rats, 4-hour exposure (Decis PM 2.5 percent), Huntingdon Research Centre, (Unpublished report RSL 437/80568, submitted to WHO by Roussel Uclaf).

COOMBS, D.W. & CLARK, G.C. (1978) RU 22974: Acute inhalation toxicity in rats. 6 Hour $LC_{50}$. Huntingdon, Huntingdon Research Centre, (Unpublished report RSL 310/78453/A, submitted to WHO by Roussel Uclaf).

COOMBS, D.W., CLARK, G.C., STREET, A.E., & GIBSON, W.A. (1978) RU 22974 inhalation toxicity study in rats 14 x 6 hour exposures over a period of 3 weeks (Unpublished proprietary report RSL/318/78638/A, submitted to WHO by Roussel Uclaf).

COQUET, B. (1976a) RU 22974. Test to determine primary cutaneous irritation in the rabbit. Joinville-le-Pont, Institut Français de Recherches et Essais Biologiques (Unpublished report IFREB-R 761157/A, submitted by Roussel Uclaf to WHO).

COQUET, B. (1976b) RU 22974. Test to evaluate ocular irritation in the rabbit, Joinville-le-Pont, Institut Français de Recherches et Essais Biologiques (Unpublished report IFREB- R 761158/A, submitted to WHO by Roussel Uclaf).

COQUET, B. (1977) RU 22974. Decis formulations - Determination of the $LD_{50}$ in the rat by oral administration, Joinville-le-Pont, Institut Français de Recherches et Essais Biologiques (Unpublished report 770257-A, submitted to WHO by Roussel Uclaf).

COTONAT, J., BLEYS, M., & FOULHOUX, P. (1987) Effets antagonistes du phenprobamate et du carbamate de mephenesine sur l'intoxication a la deltaméthrine. J. Toxicol. clin. exp., **7**: 5-19.

CROFTON, K.M. & REITER, L.W. (1984) Effects of two pyrethroid insecticides on motor activity and the acoustic startle response in the rat. Toxicol. appl. Pharmacol., **75:** 318-328

DAVID, D. (1981) Laboratory evaluation of repellent properties against birds of the synthetic pyrethroid decamethrin. Poult. Sci., **60**: 1149-1151.

DAVIES, J.E., MUNT, P.L., & GOOR, J.L. (1983) RU 22974. Investigation of possible neurological effects using the tilting plane test. Huntingdon, Huntingdon Research Centre (Unpublished proprietary report RSL603/83232/A, submitted to WHO by Roussel Uclaf).

DE LAVAUR, E., LE SECH, J., & GROLLEAU, G. (1985) Accumulation et élimination de la deltaméthrine chez la caille japonaise. Ann. Fals. Exp. Chim., **835:** 73-78.

DOHERTY, J.D., LAUTER, C.J., & SALEM, N., Jr (1986) Synaptic effects of the synthetic pyrethroid resmethrin in rat brain *in vitro*. Comp. Biochem. Physiol., **C84**(2): 373-9.

DUCLOHIER, H. & GEORGESCAULD, D. (1979) The effects of the insecticide decamethrin on action potential and voltage-clamp currents of myxicola giant axon. Comp. Biochem. Physiol., **C62**(2): 217-223.

DUMONT, C. & CHIFFLOT, L. (1978) Recherche d'un antidote contre les effets toxiques aigus (Unpublished report RU-AE-72, submitted to WHO by Roussel Uclaf).

DUMONT, C. & LAURENT, J. (1979) Recherche d'antagonistes des effets neurotoxiques aigus du RU 22 974 (Unpublished report RU-AG-35, submitted to WHO by Roussel Uclaf).

DUNNING, R.A., COOPER, J.M., WARDMAN, J.M., & WINDER, G. (1981) Susceptibility of the carabid *Pterostichus melanarius* (Illiger) to aphicide sprays applied to the sugar-beet crop. (Unpublished proprietary report UK-SOIL-F.81/A, submitted to WHO by Roussel Uclaf).

DYBALL, R.E.J. (1982) Inhibition by decamethrin and resmethrin of hormone release from the isolated rat neurohypophysis - a model mammalian neurosecretory system. Pestic. Biochem. Physiol., **17:** 42-47.

ELLIOTT, M. (1977) Synthetic pyrethroids, Washington, DC, American Chemical Society, p. 229 (ACS Symposium Series 42).

ELLIOTT, M., FARNHAN, A.W., JANES, N.F., NEEDHAM, P.H., & PULMAN, D.A. (1974) Synthetic insecticide with a new order of activity. Nature, **248:** 710-711.

ESTESEN, B.J., BUCH, N.A., & WARE, G.W. (1979) Dislodgeable insecticide residue on cotton foliage; permethrin, curacron, fenvalerate, sulprofos, decis and endosulfan. Bull. environ. Contam. Toxicol., **22:** 245-248.

EVANS, M.H. (1976) End-plate potentials in frog muscle exposed to a synthetic pyrethroid, Pestic. Biochem. Physiol., **6:** 547-550.

EVERTS, J.W., VAN FRANKENHUYZEN, K., ROMAN, B., & KOEMAN, J.H. (1983) Side effects of experimental pyrethroid applications for the control of tsetse flies in a riverine forest habitat in Africa. Arch. environ. Contam. Toxicol., **12:** 91-97.

EVERTS, J.W., KORTENHOFF, B.A., HOOGLAND, H., VLUG, H.J., JACQUE, R., & KOEMAN. J.H. (1985) Effects on man-target terrestrial arthropods of synthetic pyrethroids asked for the control of the Tsetse Fly (*Glossina* spp.) in settlement areas of the Southern Ivory Coast, Africa. Arch. environ. Contam. Toxicol., **14:** 647-650.

FAO (1982) Second Government Consultation on International Harmonization of Pesticide Registration Requirements, Rome, 11-15 October, 1982, Rome, Food and Agriculture Organization of the United Nations.

FAO/WHO (1981) 1980 Evaluations of some pesticide residues in food, Rome, Food and Agriculture Organization of the United Nations (FAO Plant Production and Protection Paper No. 26 Sup).

FAO/WHO (1982) 1981 Evaluations of some pesticide residues in food, Rome, Food and Agriculture Organization of the United Nations (FAO Plant Production and Protection Paper No. 42).

FAO/WHO (1983) 1982 Evaluations of some pesticide residues in food, Rome, Food and Agriculture Organization of the United Nations (FAO Plant Production and Protection Paper No. 49).

FAO/WHO (1985a) 1984 Evaluations of some pesticide residues in food, Rome, Food and Agriculture Organization of the United Nations (FAO Plant Production and Protection Paper No. 67).

FAO/WHO (1985b) Guide to Codex recommendations concerning pesticide residues. Part 8. Recommendations for methods of analysis of pesticide residues, 3rd ed., Rome, Food and Agriculture Organization of the United Nations, Codex Committee on Pesticide Residues.

FAO/WHO (1986a) 1985 Evaluations of some pesticide residues in food. Part I - Residues, Rome, Food and Agriculture Organization of the United Nations (FAO Plant Production and Protection Paper No. 72/1).

FAO/WHO (1986b) 1986 Evaluations of some pesticide residues in food. Part I - Residues, Rome, Food and Agriculture Organization of the United Nations (FAO Plant Production and Protection Paper No. 78).

FAO/WHO (1986c) Codex maximum limits for pesticide residues, 2nd ed., Rome, Food and Agriculture Organization of the United Nations, Codex Alimentarius Commission, CAC XIII.

FAO/WHO, (1988a) 1987 Evaluations of some pesticide residues in food. Part I - Residues, Rome, Food and Agriculture Organization of the United Nations (FAO Plant Production and Protection Paper No. 86/1).

FAO/WHO, (1988b) 1988 Evaluations of some pesticide residues in food. Part 1 - residues, Rome, Food and Agriculture Organization of the United Nations. (FAO Plant Production and Protection Paper 93/1.

FAO/WHO, (1988c) Supplement 1 to Codex maximum limits for pesticide residues, Rome, Food and Agriculture Organization of the United Nations.

FISCHER, L. & CHAMBON, J.P. (1987) Faunistical inventory of cereal arthropods after flowering and incidence of insecticide treatments with deltamethrin, dimethoate and phosalone on the apigeal fauna. Meded. Fac. Landbouwwet. Rijksuniv. Gent, **52**(2a):

FLANNIGAN, S.A. & TUCKER, S.B. (1985) Variation in cutaneous sensation between synthetic pyrethroid insecticides. Contact Dermatitis, **13**: 140-147.

FLORELLI, F., GARNIER, P., & ROA, L. (1987a) Bilan de 8 années d'expérimentation sur la sélectivité du Decis vis à vis des abeilles - La défense des végétaux, **243**: 8

FLORELLI, F., HELLER, J.J., GARNIER, P., & BAUMEISTER, R. (1987b) Incidence sur les abeilles, les ruches et leur production, de traitements aériens du colza avec la deltaméthrine - Annales ANPP - Conférence Internationale sur les Ravageurs en Agriculture, Paris, 1-3 décembre 1987, 189-203.

FORSHAW, P.J. & BRADBURY, J.E. (1983) Pharmacological effects of pyrethroids on the cardiovascular system of the rat. Eur. J. Pharmacol., **91**: 207-213.

FORSHAW, P.J. & RAY, D.E. (1986) The effects of two pyrethroids, cismethrin and deltamethrin, on skeletal muscle and the trigeminal reflex system in the rat. Pestic. Biochem. Physiol., **25**: 143-151.

FORSHAW, P.J., LISTER, T., & RAV, D.E. (1987) The effects of two types of pyrethroid on rat skeletal muscle. Eur. J. Pharmacol., **134**(1): 89-96.

FOUILLET, X. (1976) RU 22974 Mutagenicity study of various preparations. *Salmonella* microsome test, Institut Francais de Recherches et Essais Biologiques (Unpublished report no. IFREB-R 761153/A, submitted to WHO by Roussel Uclaf).

FOULHOUX, P. (1981) Medical observations of personnel working on synthesis or formulation of deltamethrin (Unpublished report RU-81.18.06/A, submitted to WHO by Roussel Uclaf).

FOULHOUX, P. (1988) Assessment of potential adverse effects of deltamethrin on man, Département Central de Toxicovigilance Roussel Uclaf, 16 pp. (Unpublished report submitted to WHO by Roussel Uclaf).

FOULHOUX, P., BOGGIN, CORNILLIET, POTTIER, RAYNAUD, STERN-VEYRIN, & SUTTET (1981) Cutaneous irritation patch test on human volunteers with Decis EC25, Decis flowable 25, Decis + mineral oil 25 (Unpublished report RU-81.03.02/DM/A, submitted to WHO by Roussel Uclaf).

FOURNIER, P.E. (1988) Etude de l'activité antidote du carbamate d'éthyl dans l'intoxication aiguë par la deltaméthrine chez le rat, Paris, Unit de Pharmacologie Clinique, Hospital Fernand Widal (Unpublished report submitted to WHO by Roussel Uclaf).

GAINES, T.B. & LINDER, R.E. (1986) Acute toxicity of pesticides in adult and weanling rats, Fundam. appl. Toxicol., **7**: 299-308.

GAMMON, D.W. & CASIDA, J.E. (1983) Pyrethroids of the most potent class antagonize GABA action at the crayfish neuromuscular junction. Neurosci. Lett., **40**: 163-168.

GAMMON, D.W., BROWN, M.A., & CASIDA, J.E. (1981) Two classes of pyrethroid action in the cockroach. Pestic. Biochem. Physiol., **15**: 181-191.

GAMMON, D.W., LAWRENCE, L.J., & CASIDA, J.E. (1982) Pyrethroid toxicology: Protective effects of diazepam and phenobarbital in the mouse and the cockroach. Toxicol. appl. Pharmacol., **66**: 290-296.

GLICKMAN, A.H. & CASIDA, J.E. (1982) Species and structural variations affecting pyrethroid neurotoxicity. Neurobehav. Toxicol. Teratol., **4**(6): 793-799.

GLOMOT, R. (1979) Acute toxicity study by oral route in the rat (Proprietary report RU-79803-54/A2, submitted to WHO by Roussel Uclaf).

GLOMOT, R. & CHEVALIER, B. (1976a) RU 22974. Acute toxicity study mouse and rat by oral route (Unpublished report TOX 76810/A, submitted to WHO by Roussel Uclaf).

GLOMOT, R. & CHEVALIER, B. (1976b) RU 22974. Acute toxicity study mouse and rat by intraperitoneal route (Unpublished report TOX 76811/A, submitted to WHO by Roussel Uclaf).

GLOMOT, R. & CHEVALIER, B. (1976c) RU 22974. Acute toxicity study mouse and rat by intravenous route (Unpublished report TOX 76812/A, submitted to WHO by Roussel Uclaf).

GLOMOT, R. & VANNIER, B. (1977) RU 22974. Teratological study in mouse, rat and rabbit (Unpublished report TOX 76534-76536/2/A, submitted to WHO by Roussel Uclaf).

GLOMOT, R. & VANNIER, B. (1978) RU 22974. Teratological study in rabbit. Complementary information (Unpublished report TOX 76534-76536/A3, submitted to WHO by Roussel Uclaf).

GLOMOT, R., AUDEGOND, L., & COLLAS, E. (1979) Acute oral toxicity study in the rat (Decis 25 G/L Mixofluid) (Proprietary report RU 79824/A, submitted to WHO by Roussel Uclaf).

GLOMOT, R., AUDEGOND, L., & COLLAS, E. (1980a) Single administration by oral route in the mouse (Decis Wettable Powder, 2.5%) (Proprietary report RU-80817/A, submitted to WHO by Roussel Uclaf).

GLOMOT, R., AUDEGOND, L., & COLLAS, E. (1980b) Single administration study by oral route in the dog (Decis Wettable Powder, 2.5%) (Proprietary report RU 80194/A, submitted to WHO by Roussel Uclaf).

GLOMOT, R., AUDEGOND, L., & COLLAS, E. (1981a) Single administration study by oral route in the rat (Proprietary report RU-81239/A, submitted WHO by Roussel Uclaf).

GLOMOT, R., AUDEGOND, L., & COLLAS, E. (1981b) Primary dermal irritation study in the rabbit. Deltamethrin 25 G/L Mixofluid (Proprietary report RU-79193/A, submitted to WHO by Roussel Uclaf).

GLOMOT, R., AUDEGOND, L., & COLLAS, E. (1981c) Primary dermal irritation study in the rabbit (Deltamethrin wettable powder, 2.5%) (Proprietary report RU-80200/A, submitted to WHO by Roussel Uclaf).

GLOMOT, R., AUDEGOND, L., & COLLAS, E. (1981d) Primary eye irritation study in the rabbit (Deltamethrin in 25 G/L Mixofluid) (Proprietary report RU-79192/A, submitted to WHO by Roussel Uclaf).

GLOMOT, R., AUDEGOND, L., & COLLAS., E. (1981e) Primary eye irritation study in the rabbit (Decis Wettable Powder, 2.5%) (Proprietary report RU-79192/A, submitted WHO by Roussel Uclaf).

GLOMOT, R., CHEVALIER, B., COLLAS, E., & AUDEGOND, L. (1977) RU 22974. Acute toxicity study by oral route in male and female Beagle dogs (Unpublished report TOX 77804/JL-5, submitted to WHO by Roussel Uclaf).

GOLDENTHAL, E.I., BLAIR, M., JEFFERSON, N.D., SPICER, E.J.F., ARCEO, R.J., & KAHN, A., III (1980a) RU 22974. Two year toxicity and carcinogenicity study in mice, Mattawan, Michigan, International Research and Development Corporation (Unpublished report IRDC 406-001/A-4, submitted to WHO by Roussel Uclaf).

GOLDENTHAL, E.I., JEFFERSON, N.D., BLAIR, M., THORSTENSON, J.H., SPICER, E.J.F., ARCEO, R.J., & KAHN, A., III (1980b) RU 22974. Two year oral toxicity and carcinogenicity study in rats, Mattawan, Michigan, International Research and Development Corporation (Unpublished report IRDC 406-002/A.4, submitted to WHO by Roussel Uclaf).

GRANDADAM, A. (1976) Test to determine the toxicity in the chicken by oral route (Unpublished report RU76.05.05/A, submitted to WHO by Roussel Uclaf).

GRAY, A.J. & RICKARD, J. (1982) The toxicokinetics of deltamethrin in rats after intravenous administration of a toxic dose. Pestic. Biochem. Physiol.., **18:** 205-215.

GRAY, A.J., CONNORS, T.A., & RICKARD, J. (1980) Mechanism of mammalian toxicity of the pyrethroids. In: Littaner, U.Z. et al., ed. Neurotransmitters and their receptors, New York, John Wiley and Sons, pp. 565-568.

GROLLEAU G. & GRIBAN, J. (1976a) Toxicity of deltamethrin or DECIS in single ingestion in game duck *Anas platyrhnchos* L., JoyenJossas, France, Institut National de la Recherche Agronomique (Unpublished report INRA-76.21 12/A, submitted to WHO by Roussel Uclaf).

GROLLEAU, G. & GRIBAN, J. (1976b) Toxicity of deltamethrin or DECIS by single ingestion in grey partridge, *Perdix Perdix* L. and red partridge, *Alectotis rufa* L., JoyenJossas, France, Institut National de la Recherche Agronomique (Unpublished report INRA76.28 09/A, submitted to WHO by Roussel Uclaf).

GUILLOT, J.P. & GUILAINE, J. (1977) RU 22974. Decaméthrine. Decis technical Roussel Uclaf. Sensitization test in the guinea pig. Joinville-le-Pont, Institut Français de Recherches et Essais Biologique (Unpublished report no. IFREB-R 709241/A, submitted to WHO by Roussel Uclaf).

GULYAS P. & CSANYI B. (undated) Acute fish toxicological investigation of diverse insecticides, Hungary, Scientific Research Centre of Economy of Water Supplies, 21 pp. (Unpublished proprietary data supplied to WHO by Roussel Uclaf).

HALLS, G.R.H. & PERIAM, A.W. (1980) The fate of residues of NRDC 161 on wheat during storage and after milling and baking - Report after 9 months storage, November 1980, Wellcome Research Laboratories Report (Unpublished report HEFH 80-4, submitted to WHO by Roussel Uclaf).

HARGREAVES, J.R. & COOPER, L.P. (1979) Phytotoxicity tests with pyrethroid insecticides on glasshouse grown tomato seedlings. Queensland J. Agric. anim. Sci., **36:** 151-154.

HASCOET, M. (1977) Laboratory leaching soil study with decamethrin (RU 22974), Versailles, Institut National de la Recherche Agronomique (Unpublished proprietary report INRA-77.20.09/A, submitted to WHO by Roussel Uclaf).

HE, F. (1987) Occupational neurotoxicology: Current problems and trends. Paper presented at the XXII International Congress on Occupational Health, Sydney, 27 September-2 October, 1987.

HE, F., WANG, S., LIU, L., CHEN, S., ZHANG, Z., & SUN, J. (1989) Clinical manifestations and diagnosis of acute pyrethroid poisoning. Arch. Toxicol., **63**: 54-58.

HEHEITMULLER, T., SHUBA, P.J., & PARRISH, R. (1978) Acute toxicity of Decis to sheepshead minnows (*Cyprinodon variegatus*), E.G. & G. Bionomics Marine Laboratory, 7 pp. (Unpublished proprietary report BR-78-12219, supplied to WHO by Roussel Uclaf).

HEWSON, R.T. & BURGESS, J.E. (1981) An operator study with deltamethrin including measurements of nerve conduction times (Unpublished proprietary report GB-NT-11.81A, submitted to WHO by Roussel Uclaf).

HILL, B.D. (1982) Determination of Deltamethrin residues in soils, Alberta, Agriculture Canada Research Station, 7 pp (Unpublished proprietary report CAN-82.12.10/A, submitted to WHO by Roussel Uclaf).

HILL, B.D. (1983) Persistence of deltamethrin in a Lethbridge sandy clay loam. J. environ. Sci. Health, **B18**(6): 691-703.

HILL, B.D. & JOHNSON, D.L. (1987) Persistence of deltamethrin and its isomers on pasture forage and litter. J. agric. Food Chem., **35**: 373-378.

HILL, B.D. & SCHAALJE, G.B. (1985) A two-compartment model for the dissipation of deltamethrin on soil. J. agric. food Chem., **33**: 1001-1006.

HIROMORI, T., NAKANISHI, T., KAWAGUCHI, S., SAKO, H., SUZUKI, T., & KIYAMOTO, J. (1986) Therapeutic effects of methocarbamol on acute intoxication by pyrethroids in rats. J. pestic. Sci., **11**: 9-14.

HUNTER, B., JORDAN, J., HEYWOOD, R., HEPWORTH, P., STREET, A.E., & PRENTICE, D.E. (1977) RU 22974. Assessment of toxicity to rats by oral administration for 13 weeks (followed by a 4-week withdrawal period) (Unpublished report RSL-254/76938/A3, submitted to WHO by Roussel Uclaf).

HUSSON, J.M. (1978) Medical observations made on people working on the manufacture and formulation of the pyrethroid insecticide decamethrin (Unpublished report RU 78.25.08/A, submitted to WHO by Roussel Uclaf).

IRDC (1980) Two year chronic dog feeding study, Matawan, Michigan, International Research and Development Corporation (Unpublished proprietary report IRDC-406-004/AI, submitted to WHO by Roussel Uclaf).

JACKSON, G. & HARDY, C. (1986) RU 22974. Acute inhalation toxicity in rats 1-hour exposure (Unpublished report RSL-DTM-851457/A, submitted to WHO by Roussel Uclaf).

JACQUES, Y., ROMEY, G., CAVEY, M.T., KARTAALOVSKI, B., & LAZDUNSKI, M. (1980) Interaction of pyrethroids with the sodium channel in mammalian neuronal cells in culture. Biochem. Biophys. Acta, **600**: 882-897.

KAGAN, YU. S., PANSHINA, T.N., & SASINOVICH, L.M. (1986) Biochemical effects of toxic action of synthetic pyrethroids. Gig. i Sanit., 1: 7-9.

KAUFMAN, D.D. & KAYSER, A.J. (1979a) Degradation of $^{14}$C-phenoxy- and $^{14}$C-cyano-decamethrin in soil (Unpublished proprietary report USDA-I-23.04.79/A2, submitted to WHO by Roussel Uclaf).

KAUFMAN, D.D. & KAYSER, A.J. (1979b) The effect of soil temperature on the degradation of $^{14}$C-cyano-decamethrin in soil (Unpublished proprietary report USDA-II-24.04.79/A2, submitted to WHO by Roussel Uclaf).

KAUFMAN, D.D. & KAYSER, A.J. (1980) Degradation of $^{14}$C-cyano-, $^{14}$C-phenoxy-, and $^{14}$C-vinyl-decamethrin in flooded soil (Unpublished proprietary report USDA-III-12.05.80/A, submitted to WHO by Roussel Uclaf).

KAUFMAN, D.D., RUSSEL, B.A., HELLING, C.S., & KAYSER, A.J. (1981) Movement of cypermethrin, decamethrin, permethrin and their degradation products in soil. J. agric. food Chem., **29**: 239-245.

KAVLOCK, R., CHERNOFF, N., BARON, R., LINDER, R., ROGERS, E., CARVER, B., DILLEY, J., & SIMMON, V. (1979) Toxicity studies with decamethrin, a synthetic pyrethroid insecticide. J. environ. Pathol. Toxicol., **2**: 751-765.

KNAUF, W. & HORLEIN, G. (1979 The acute toxicity of decamethrine to the Rainbow trout *Salmo gairdneri*, Richardson, Frankfurt, Hoechst AG, 19 pp (Unpublished proprietary report 19/79, submitted to WHO by Roussel Uclaf).

KNAUF, W. & SCHULZE, E.F. (1977a) Effect of decamethrine on *Cyprinus carpio*, Frankfurt, Hoechst AG, 9 pp (Unpublished proprietary report 15/77, submitted to WHO by Roussel Uclaf).

KNAUF, W. & SCHULZE, E.F. (1977b) The effect of decamethrin 6E0660 on Catfish (*Ictalurus nebulosus*) in a static test, Frankfurt, Hoechst AG, 18 pp (Unpublished proprietary report 32/79, submitted to WHO by Roussel Uclaf).

KRASNJIH, A. & PAVLOVA, L. (1985) Harmful effects of deltamethrin. In: Levina, E., ed. Harmful substances in industry, Moscow, Khimija Publishing House, p. 154.

KYNOCH, S.R., LLOYD, G.K., & ANDREWS, C.D. (1979) Acute percutaneous toxicity to rats of decamethrin, Huntingdon, Huntingdon Research Centre (Unpublished report RSL-1009 8/D, submitted to WHO by Roussel Uclaf).

LAWRENCE, L.J. & CASIDA, J.E. (1982) Pyrethroid toxicology: Mouse intracerebral structure-toxicity relationship. Pestic. Biochem. Physiol., **18**: 9-14.

LAWRENCE, L.J. & CASIDA, J.E. (1983) Stereospecific action of pyrethroid insecticides on the gamma-aminobutyric acid receptor-ionophore complex. Science, **221:** 1399-1401.

LAWRENCE, L.J., GEE, K.W., & YAMAMURA, H.I. (1985) Interactions of pyrethroid insecticides with chloride ionophore-associated binding sites. Neurotoxicology, **6:** 87-98.

LEAHEY, J.P. (1985) The pyrethroid insecticide, London, Taylor & Francis Ltd., p. 440.

LECLERCQ, M., COTONAT, J., & FOULHOUX, P. (1986) Recherche d'un antagoniste à l'intoxication par la deltaméthrine. J. Toxicol. clin. exp., **6,** 83-85.

LEIBOWITZ, M.D., SCHWARZ, J.R., HOLAN, G., & HILLE, B. (1987) Electrophysiological comparison of insecticide and alkaloid agonists of Na channels. J. gen. Physiol., **90**(1): 75-93.

LEPAILLEUR, H. & CHAMBON, A. (1984) Etude de la toxicité létale du produit technique deltaméthrine vis à vis du poisson-zebré, 5 pp. (Unpublished proprietary dated report IRCHA B.7827, submitted to WHO by Roussel Uclaf).

LHOSTE, J., FRANCOIS, Y., & RUPAUD, Y. (1979) Ichtyotoxicité de la decaméthrine vis à vis de *Salmo trutta* L. (poisson téléostéen) en fonction de l'age et des conditions expérimentales - Congrès sur la lutte contre les insectes en milieu tropical, Marseilles - March 13-16 1979, pp. 885-902.

L'HOTELLIER, M. & VINCENT, P. (1986) Assessment of the impact of deltamethrin on aquatic species. In British Crop Protection Conference - Pests and Disease: 1109-1116.

LOUVEAUX, J., MISSONNIER, J., & MESQUIDA, J. (1977) Tests de toxicité sur abeille domestique avec le Decis CE (Unpublished proprietary report submitted to WHO by Roussel Uclaf).

LUMMIS, S.C., CHOW, S.C., HOLAN, G., & JOHNSTON, G.A. (1987) Gamma-aminobutyric acid receptor ionophore complexes: differential effects of deltamethrin, dichlorodiphenyltrichloroethane, and some novel insecticides in a rat brain membrane preparation. J. Neurochem., **48**(3): 689-94.

LUND, A.E. & NARAHASHI, T. (1983) Kinetics of sodium channel modification as the basis for the variation in the nerve membrane effects of pyrethroids and DDT analogs. Pestic. Biochem. Physiol., **20:** 203-216.

MACPHAIL, R.C. (1981) Behavioral effects of a synthetic insecticide (decamethrin). Fed. Proc. Fed. Am. Soc. Exp. Biol., **40:** 678.

MEISTER, R.T., BERG, G.L., SINE, C., MEISTER, S., & POPLYK, J. (1983) Farm chemicals handbook. Section C. Pesticide dictionary, Willoughby, Ohio, Meister Publishing Co.

MESTRES, R., CHEVALLIER, C., ESPNOZA, C., & CORNET, R. (1978a) Dosage des résidus de decaméthrine dans les produits végétaux. Trav. Soc. Pharm. Montpellier, **38**: 183-192.

MESTRES R., CHEVALLIER C., & ESPINOZA, C. (1978b) Analytical method for decamethrine residue analysis, Montpellier, Faculte de Pharmacie, 2 pp. (Proprietary report FP-78.08.07/A, dated 7/8/1978 submitted to WHO by Roussel Uclaf).

MESTRES, R., FRANCOIS, C., CAUSSE C., VIAN L., & WINNETT, G. (1985) Survey of exposure to pesticides in greenhouses. Bull. environ. Contam. Toxicol., **35**: 750-756.

MESTRES, R., ESPINOZA, C., & CHEVALLIER, C. (1986) Effets sur les résidus de deltaméthrine de la transformation des produits agricoles en vue de leur consommation. Med. Nutr., XXII (**3**): 181-184.

MILLER, T.A. & ADAMS, M.E. (1980) Neural and behavioral correlates of pyrethroid and DDT-type poisoning in the housefly, *Musca domestica*. Pestic. Biochem. Physiol., **13**: 137-147.

MIYAMOTO, J. (1976) Degradation, metabolism and toxicity of synthetic pyrethroids. Environ. Health Perspect., **14**: 15-28.

MIYAMOTO, J. (1981) The chemistry, metabolism and residue analysis of synthetic pyrethroids, Pure appl. Chem., **53**: 1967-2022.

MIYAMOTO, J. & KEARNEY, P.C. (1983) Pesticide chemistry - Human welfare and the environment. Proceedings of the Fifth International Congress of Pesticide Chemistry, Kyoto, Japan, 29 August - 4 September, 1982, Oxford, Pergamon Press, Vol. 1-4.

MOHSEN, Z.H. & MULLA, M.S. (1981) Toxicity of blackfly larvicidal formulations to some aquatic insects in the laboratory. Bull. environ. Contam. Toxicol., **26**: 696-703.

MOUROT, D., DELEPINE, B., BOISSEAU, J., & GAYOT, G. (1979) High-performance liquid chromatography of decamethrin. J. Chromatogr., **173**: 412-414.

MUIR, D.C.G., RAWN, G.P., & GRIFT, N.P., (1985) Fate of the pyrethroid insecticide deltamethrin in small ponds: A mass balance study. J. agric. food Chem., **33**: 603-609.

MULLA, M.S., NAVVAB GOJRATI, H.A., & DARWAZEH, H.A. (1978) Toxicity of mosquito larvicidal pyrethroids to four species of freshwater fishes. Environ. Entomol.., **7**(3): 428-430.

NETO, P.X.R., RODRIGUES, I.C.F., & FILHO, A.M (1983) Etude sur les effets secondaires de la deltamethrine sur l'ichtyofaune de la region du projet "Rio Formoso" (Unpublished report submitted to WHO by Roussel Uclaf).

NOBLE, R.M., HAMILTON, D.J., & OSBORNE, W.J. (1982) Stability of pyrethroids on wheat in storage. Pestic. Sci., **13**: 246-252.

PANSHINA T.N. & SASINOVICH, L.M. (1983) Toxicology of synthetic pyrethroids. Khim. sel'sk. khoz., **12:** 51-53.

PANSU, M., DHOUIBI, M.H., & PINTA, M. (1981) Determination of traces of biopermethrine and decamethrine pyrethrinoids in biological substrates by gas chromatography. Analysis, **9**: 55-59.

PAPALEXIOU, Ph., BITAR, N., & STOCKIS, A. (1984) Absorption of radiocarbon labelled deltamethrin given orally in healthy volunteers, Charleroi, Belgium, Institut de Pharmacologie et d'Investigations Biomédicales (Unpublished proprietary report 50/22, submitted to WHO by Roussel Uclaf).

PARKIN, P.J. & LEQUESNE, P.M. (1982) Effects of a synthetic pyrethroid deltamethrin on excitability changes following a nerve impulse. J. Neurol. Neurosurg. Psychiatry., **45**: 337-342.

PEYRE, M., CHANTOT, J.F., GLOMOT, R., & PENASSE, L. (1980) Detection of a mutagenic potency of decamethrin (RU 22974), in bacterial tests (Unpublished report RU/TOX/80-2101/A, submitted to WHO by Roussel Uclaf).

PHAM, H.C., NAVARRO-DALMASURE, C., PHAM, H.C., CLAVEL, P., VAN HAVERBEKE, G., CHEAV, S.L. (1984) Toxicological studies of deltamethrin. Int. J. Tissue React., **6**(2): 127-33.

PICHON, Y. (1981) Pharmacological characterization of ionic channels in unmyelinated axons. J. Physiol., **17**(9): 1119-1128.

PLAPP, F.W., Jr & BULL, D.L. (1978) Toxicity and selectivity of some insecticides to Chrysopa carnea, a predator of the tobacco budworm. Environ. Entomol., **7**: 431-434.

PLESTINA, R. (1981) An evaluation of the use of deltamethrin in public health (Unpublished report ZAG. KOT. 81/A, submitted to WHO by Roussel Uclaf).

PLUIJMEN, M., DREVON, C., MONTESANO, R., MALAVEILLE C., HAUTEFEUILLE, A., & BARTSCH, H. (1984) Lack of mutagenicity of synthetic pyrethroids in *Salmonella typhimurium* strains and in V79 Chinese hamster cells. Mutat. Res., **137:** 7-15.

POLAKOVA, H. & VARGOVA, M. (1983) Evaluation of the mutagenic effects of decamethrin: cytogenetic analysis of bone marrow. Mutat. Res., **120**: 167-171.

POTTIER J., CHATELET, P., & JOUQUEY, S. (1982) Resorption percutanée de la deltaméthrine - Etude d'un modèle animal, 10 pp. (Unpublished proprietary report AN.34, submitted to WHO by Roussel Uclaf).

PRASADA RAO, K.S., CHETTY, C.S., & DESAIAH, D. (1984) *In vitro* effects of pyrethroids on rat brain and liver ATPase activities. J Toxicol. environ. Health, **14**(2-3): 257-65.

RAWN, G.P., MUIR, D.O.G., & GRIFT, P.G. (1985) Fate of the pyrethroid insecticide deltamethrin in small ponds, a mass balance study. J. agr. food Chem., **33:** 603-609.

RAY, D.E. (1980) An EEG investigation of decamethrin-induced choreathetosis in the rat. Exp. Brain Res., **38**: 221-227.

RAY, D.E. (1982) Changes in brain blood flow associated with deltamethrin-induced choreoathetosis in the rat. Exp. Brain Res., **45**: 269-276.

RAY, D.E. & CREMER, J.E. (1979) The action of decamethrin (a synthetic pyrethroid) on the rat. Pestic. Biochem. Physiol., **10**: 333-340.

RICHTER, W.R. & GOLDENTHAL, E.I. (1983) Two-year oral toxicity and carcinogenicity study in rats. Amendment to the final report. Matawan, Michinga, International Research and Development Corporation (Unpublished proprietary report IRDC 406.002/A5, submitted to WHO by Roussel Uclaf).

RICKARD, J. & BRODIE, M.E. (1985) Correlation of blood and brain levels of the neurotoxic pyrethroid deltamethrin with the onset of symptoms in rats. Pestic. Biochem. Physiol., **23**: 143-156.

RICOU (1978) Assessment of side effects of S 276-B (Decis EC 25 g/l) towards grey slugs (*Agriolimax* spp.) (Unpublished proprietary report INRA-LIM.78.10/A, submitted to WHO by Roussel Uclaf).

ROSE, G.P. & DEWAR, A.J. (1983) Intoxication with four synthetic pyrethroids fail to show any correlation between neuromuscular dysfunction and neurobiochemical abnormalities in rats. Arch. Toxicol., **53**: 297-316.

ROSE, D.B., ROBERTS, N.L., CAMERON, M.McD., PRENTICE, D.E., COOKE, L., & GIBSON, W.A. (1978) RU 22974. (Decamethrine) $LD_{50}$ determination and assessment of neurotoxicity in the domestic hen, Huntingdon, Huntingdon Research Centre (Unpublished report RSL 293-NT/7830/A, submitted to WHO by Roussel Uclaf).

ROUSSELIN, X. (1983) Toxicité des dérivés du pyrèthre, Paris, Faculté de Médecine Lariboisiere-Saint-Louis (Thèse de l'Université Paris VII).

RUIGT, G.S.F. & VAN DEN BERCKEN, J. (1986) Action of pyrethroids on a nerve-muscle preparation of the clawed frog, *Xenopus laevis*. Pestic. Biochem. Physiol., **25**: 176-187.

RUZO, L.O. & CASIDA, J.E. (1979) Degradation of decamethrin on cotton plants. J. agric. food Chem., **27**: 572-575.

RUZO, L.O., HOLMSTEAD, R.L., & CASIDA, J.E. (1976) Solution photochemistry of the potent pyrethroid insecticide α-cyano-3-phenoxybenzyl *cis*-2,2-dimethyl-3-(2,2-dibromovinyl)cyclopropanecarboxylate. Tetrahedron Lett., 3045-3048.

RUZO, L.O., HOLMSTEAD, R.L., & CASIDA, J.E. (1977) Pyrethroid photochemistry: decamethrin. J. agric. food Chem., **25**: 1385-1394.

RUZO, L.O., UNAI, T., & CASIDA, J.E. (1978) Decamethrin metabolism in rats. J. agric. food Chem., **26**: 918-925.

RUZO, L.O., ENGEL, J.L., & CASIDA, J.E. (1979) Decamethrin metabolites from oxidative, hydrolytic and conjugative reactions in mice. J. agric. food Chem., **27**: 725-731.

SANTOSA, K. (1983) Toxicity of Decis 2.5 EC (Decamethrin) to fish, Jakarta, Department of Agriculture Research and Development Inland Fisheries Institute, 4 pp. (Unpublished proprietary data submitted to WHO by Roussel Uclaf).

SANTOSA, K. & HADI, H. (1980) Trial results pesticide lethal toxicity to fish, Department of Agriculture Research and Development Inland Fisheries Institute, Jakarta, Indonesia - Report no. 174/UI/80 dated 5 December 1980, 3 pp. (Unpublished proprietary data submitted to WHO by Roussel Uclaf).

SMIES, M., EVERS, R.H.J., REIJNENBURG, P.H.M., & KOEMAN, J.H. (1980) Environmental aspects of field trials with pyrethroids to eradicate tsetse fly in Nigeria. Ecotoxicol. environ. Saf., **4**: 114-128.

SOBELS, F.H., TATES, A.D., & VANNIER, B. (1978) Cytogenetic study with RU 22974. Detection of a mutagenic potency in mammalian cells, Leiden, The Netherlands, State University of Leiden (Unpublished report ULN-782211/A, submitted to WHO by Roussel Uclaf).

SODERLUND, D.M. & CASIDA, J.E. (1977) Effects of pyrethroid structure on rates of hydrolysis and oxidation by mouse liver microsomal enzymes. Pestic. Biochem. Physiol., **7**: 391-401.

SOUYRI, F. (1985) Autoradiographic studies of ($^3$H)-deltamethrin binding with nerve tissue cultures. Pestic. Sci., **6**(6): 701-703.

STAATZ, C.G., BLOOM, A.S., & LECH, J.J. (1982) Effects of pyrethroids on [3H]-kainic acid binding to mouse forebrain membranes. Toxicol. appl. Pharmacol., **64**: 566-569.

STAATZ-BENSON, C.G. & HOSKO, M.J. (1986) Interaction of pyrethroids with mammalian spinal neurons. Pestic. Biochem. Physiol., **25**: 19-30.

STEIN, E.A., WASHBURN, M., WALCZAK, C., & BLOOM, A.S. (1987) Effects of pyrethroid insecticides on operant responding maintained by food. Neurotoxicol. Teratol., **9**(1): 27-31.

STEVENSON, J.H., NEEDHAM, P.H., & WALKER, J. (1978) Poisoning of honey bee by pesticides: investigations of the changing pattern in Britain over 20 years. Rothamsted Exp. Stn Rep., Part 2: 55-72.

TAKAHASHI, M. & LEQUESNE, P. ((1982) The effects of the pyrethroids deltamethrin and cismethrin on nerve excitability in rats. J. Neurol. Neurosurg. Psychiatry, **45**: 1005-1011.

TAKKEN, W., BALK, F., JANSEN, R.C., & KOEMAN, J.H. (1978) The experimental application of insecticides from a helicopter for the control of riverine populations of *Glossina tachinoides* in West Africa. VI. Observations on side effects. P.A.N.S., **24**: 455-466.

THIEBAULT, J.J., BOST, J., & FOULHOUX, P. (1985) Intoxication expérimentale par la deltaméthrine chez le chien et son traitement. Toxicol. vét. Collect. Méd. lég. Toxicol. méd., **131,** 47-62.

THIEBAULT, J.J., BOST, J., FOULHOUX, P., DEVAUX, P., & TILLIER, C. (in press) Intravenous deltamethrin intoxication of dogs. Therapeutic attempts. Veterinary and Human Toxicology.

THIER, W. & SCHMIDT, D. (1976) Laboratory leaching studies of Decis EC 25 in three different German soils (Unpublished proprietary report RL-77.25.05/A, submitted to WHO by Roussel Uclaf).

THIER, W. & SCHMIDT, D. (1977) [Verhalten des Pflanzenschutzmittelwirkstoffes im Boden: Decamethrin], (Unpublished proprietary report A09232, submitted to WHO by Roussel Uclaf) (in German).

TONG YING (1988) Clinical manifestations of 211 cases intoxicated by deltamethrin and fenvalerate (Unpublished report submitted to WHO by Roussel Uclaf).

TOOBY, T.E., THOMSON, A.N., RYCROFT, R.J., BLACK, I.A., & HEWSON, R.T. (1981) A pond study to investigate the effects on fish and aquatic invertebrates of deltamethrin applied directly onto water, Fisheries Laboratory, Ministry of Agriculture, Fisheries and Food (Unpublished report AEP-81.30.09A, submitted to WHO by Roussel Uclaf).

TRIVEDI, K. (1981) Spray worker exposure and health survey during decamethrin (decis) spray in the field, Sevagram, India, Mahatma Gandhi Institute of Medical Sciences (Unpublished information submitted to WHO by Roussel Uclaf).

TU, C.M. (1980) Influence of five pyrethroid insecticides on microbial populations and activities in soil. Microb. Ecol., **5:** 321-327.

VAN DEN BERCKEN, J. (l977) The action of allethrin on the peripheral nervous system of the frog. Pestic. Sci., **8:** 692-699.

VAN DEN BERCKEN, J. & VIJVERBERG, H.P.M. (1980) Voltage clamp studies on the effects of allethrin and DDT on the sodium channels in frog myelinated nerve membrane. In: Insect neurobiology and pesticide action (Neutox 79), London, Society of Chemical Industry, Vol. 2, pp. 79-85.

VAN DEN BERCKEN, J., AKKERMANS, L.M.A., & VAN DER ZALM, J.M. (1973) DDT-like action of allethrin in the sensory nervous system of *Xenopus laevis*. Eur. J. Pharmacol., **21**: 95-106.

VAN DEN BERCKEN, J., KROESE, A.B.A., & AKKERMANS, L.M.A. (1979) Effect of insecticides on the sensory nervous system. In: Narahashi, T., ed. Neurotoxicology of insecticides and pheromones, New York, London, Plenum Press, pp. 183-210.

VANNIER, B. & FOURNEX, R. (1983) Deltamethrin detection of a mutagenic potency/micronucleus test in the mouse (Proprietary unpublished report RU-83607/A, submitted to WHO by Roussel Uclaf).

VANNIER, B. & GLOMOT, R. (1977) RU 22974. Mutagenic study. Dominant lethal assay in the male mouse (Unpublished report TOX 76533/DB9/A, submitted to WHO by Roussel Uclaf).

VANNIER, B. & GLOMOT, R. (1982) RU 22974 complementary teratological study in the mouse (Unpublished report RU-82506-12/A, submitted to WHO by Roussel Uclaf).

VARANKA, I. (1987) Effect of mosquito killer insecticides on freshwater mussels. Comp. Biochem. Physiol. C. Comp. Pharmacol., **86**: 157-162.

VAYSSE, M., GIUDICELLI, J.C., DEVAUX, P., & L'HOTELLIER, M. (1984) Decis, in Zweig analytical methods for pesticides and plant growth regulators. Vol XIII, **3**: 53-68, New York, Academic Press.

VERSCHOYLE, R.D. & ALDRIDGE, W.N. (1980) Structure-activity relationship of some pyrethroids in rats. Arch. Toxicol., **45**: 325-329.

VICKERMAN, G.P., COOMBES D.S., TURNER, G., MEAD-BRIGGS, M.A., & EDWARDS, J. (1987a) The effects of pirimicarb, dimethoate and deltamethrin on Carabidae and Staphylinidae in winter wheat. Meded. Fac. Landbouwwet. Rijksuniv. Gent, **52**(2a):

VICKERMAN, G.P., COOMBES, D.S., TURNER, G., MEAD-BRIGGS, M.A., & EDWARDS, J. (1987b) The effects of pirimicarb, dimethoate and deltamethrin on non-target arthropods in winter wheat. International Conference on Pests in Agriculture, Paris, 1-3 December 1987, Annales ANPP, pp. 67-74.

VIJVERBERG, H.P.M., VAN DEN BECKEN, J. (1982) Action of pyrethroid insecticides on the vertebrate nervous system. Neuropathol. appl. Neurobiol., **8**: 421-440.

VIJVERBERG, H.P.M. & VAN DEN BERCKEN, J. (1979) Frequency dependent effects of the pyrethroid insecticide decamethrin in frog myelinated nerve fibres. Eur. J. Pharmacol., **58**: 501-504.

VIJVERBERG, H.P.M., RUIGT, G.S.F., & VAN DEN BERCKEN, J. (1982a) Structure-related effects of pyrethroid insecticides on the lateral-line sense organ and on peripheral nerves of the clawed frog, *Xenopus laevis*. Pestic. Biochem. Physiol., **18**: 315-324.

VIJVERBERG, H.P.M., VAN DER ZALM, J.M., & VAN DEN BERCKEN, J. (1982b) Similar mode of action of pyrethroids and DDT on sodium channel gating in myelinated nerves. Nature, (Lond.) **295**: 601-603.

VIJVERBERG, H.P.M., VAN DER ZALM, J.M., VAN KLEEF, R.G.D.M., & VAN DEN BERCKEN, J. (1983) Temperature and structure-dependent interaction of pyrethroids with the sodium channels in frog node of Ranvier. Biochim. Biophys. Acta, **728**: 73-82.

WALTERSDORFER & SCHULZE E.F. (1976a) Decis 2.5. Effect on *Lebistes reticulatus*, Frankfurt, Hoechst AG, 8 pp. (Unpublished proprietary report 42/76, submitted to WHO by Roussel Uclaf).

WALTERSDORFER & SCHULZE E.F. (1976b) Decis 2.5. Effect on *Idus melanotus,* Frankfurt, Hoechst AG, 5 pp (Unpublished proprietary report 33/76, submitted to WHO by Roussel Uclaf).

WALTERSDORFER & SCHULZE E.F. (1976c) Decis 2.5. Effect on *Salmo gairdneri* (rainbow trout), Frankfurt, Hoechst AG, 7 pp (Unpublished proprietary report 35/76, submitted to WHO by Roussel Uclaf).

WALTERSDORFER & SCHULZE E.F. (1976d) Decamethrine effect on *Lepomis gibbosus* (Bluegill sunfish), Frankfurt, Hoechst AG, 6 pp. (Unpublished proprietary report 16/77, submitted to WHO by Roussel Uclaf).

WANG, S., ZHENG, Q., YU, L., XU, B., & LIX., Y. (1988) Health survey among farmers exposed to deltamethrin in the cotton fields. Ecotoxicol. environ. Saf., **15**: 1-6.

WELLCOME FOUNDATION (1979) Residues in cow's milk resulting from intrarumenal, and later, dermal administration of $^{14}$C-labelled decamethrin (Unpublished report submitted to WHO by Roussel Uclaf).

WHO (1979) Safe use of pesticides. Third Report of the WHO Expert Committee on Vector Biology and Control, Geneva, World Health Organization, pp. 18-23. (WHO Technical Report Series, No. 634).

WHO (1988) The WHO recommended classification of pesticides by hazard and guidelines to classification 1988-1989, Geneva, World Health Organization (Unpublished document WHO/VBC/88.953).

WHO (1989) Health and Safety Guide No. 30: Deltamethrin, Geneva, World Health Organization.

WHO (1984) Data sheet on pesticides, No. 50: Deltamethrin, Geneva, World Health Organization, 9 pp (Unpublished document VBC/DS/84.50).

WOOD MACKENZIE (1980) Agrochem. Monit., **9**: 12.

WOOD MACKENZIE (1981) Agrochem. Monit., **15**: 12.

WOOD MACKENZIE (1982) Agrochem. Monit., **21**: 13.

WOOD MACKENZIE (1983) Agrochem. Monit., **27**: 3-12.

WORTHING, C.R. & WALKER, S.B. (1983) Pesticide manual, 7th ed., Croydon, British Crop Protection Council, p. 161.

WOUTERS, W. & VAN DEN BERCKEN, J. (1978) Action of pyrethroids. Gen. Pharmacol., **9**: 387-398.

WRENN, J.M., RODWELL, D.E., GOLDENTHAL, E.I., SPIDER, E.J.C., & RAJASEKARAN, D. (1980) Three-generation reproduction study in rats, Matawan, Michigan, International Research and Development Corporation (Unpublished report IDC-406 003/A4. submitted to WHO by Roussel Uclaf).

ZHANG, L.Z., KHAN, S.U., AKHTAR, M.H., & IVARSON, K.C. (1984) Persistence, degradation, and distribution of Deltamethrin in an organic soil under laboratory conditions, J. agric. food Chem., **32**: 1207-1211

ZITKO, V., MCLEESE, D.W., METCALFE, C.D., & CARSON, W.G. (1979) Toxicity of permethrin, decamethrin, and related pyrethroids to salmon and lobster. Bull. environ. Contam. Toxicol., **21**: 338-343.

# APPENDIX I

On the basis of electrophysiological studies with peripheral nerve preparations of frogs (*Xenopus laevis; Rana temporaria*; and *Rana esculenta*), it is possible to distinguish between 2 classes of pyrethroid insecticides: (Type I and Type II). A similar distinction between these 2 classes of pyrethroids has been made on the basis of the symptoms of toxicity in mammals and insects (Van den Bercken et al., 1979; WHO, 1979; Verschoyle & Aldridge, 1980; Glickman & Casida, 1982; Lawrence & Casida, 1982). The same distinction was found in studies on cockroaches (Gammon et al., 1981).

Based on the binding assay on the gamma-aminobutyric acid (GABA) receptor-ionophore complex, synthetic pyrethroids can also be classified into two types: the α-cyano-3-phenoxybenzyl pyrethroids and the non-cyano pyrethroids (Gammon et al., 1982; Gammon & Casida, 1983; Lawrence & Casida, 1983; Lawrence et al., 1985).

## Pyrethroids that do not contain an α-cyano group (allethrin, d-phenothrin, permethrin, tetramethrin, cismethrin, and bioresmethrin) (Type I: T-syndrome)

The pyrethroids that do not contain an α-cyano group give rise to pronounced repetitive activity in sense organs and in sensory nerve fibres (Van den Bercken et al., 1973). At room temperature, this repetitive activity usually consists of trains of 3–10 impulses and occasionally up to 25 impulses. Train duration is between 10 and 5 milliseconds.

These compounds also induce pronounced repetitive firing of the presynaptic motor nerve terminal in the neuromuscular junction (Van den Bercken, 1977). There was no significant effect of the insecticide on neurotransmitter release, on the sensitivity of the subsynaptic membrane, or on the muscle fibre membrane. Presynaptic repetitive firing was also observed in the sympathetic ganglion treated with these pyrethroids.

In the lateral-line sense organ and in the motor nerve terminal, but not in the cutaneous touch receptor or in sensory nerve fibres, the pyrethroid-induced repetitive activity increases dramatically as the temperature is lowered, and a decrease of 5 °C in temperature may cause a more than 3-fold increase in the number of repetitive impulses per train. This effect is easily reversed by raising the temperature. The origin of this "negative temperature coefficient" is not clear (Vijverberg et al., 1983).

Synthetic pyrethroids act directly on the axon through interference with the sodium channel gating mechanism that underlies the generation and conduction of each nerve impulse. The transitional state of the sodium channel is controlled by 2 separately acting gating mechanisms, referred to as the activation gate and the inactivation gate. Since pyrethroids only appear to affect the sodium current during depolarization, the rapid opening of the activation gate and the slow closing of the inactivation gate proceed normally. However, once the sodium channel is open, the activation gate is restrained in the open position by the pyrethroid molecule. While all pyrethroids have essentially the same basic mechanism of action, however, the rate of relaxation differs substantially for the various pyrethroids (Flannigan & Tucker, 1985).

In the isolated node of Ranvier, allethrin causes prolongation of the transient increase in sodium permeability of the nerve membrane during excitation (Van den Bercken & Vijverberg, 1980). Evidence so far available indicates that allethrin selectively slows down the closing of the activation gate of a fraction of the sodium channels that open during depolarization of the membrane. The time constant of closing of the activation gate in the allethrin-affected channels is about 100 milliseconds compared with less than 100 microseconds in the normal sodium channel, i.e., it is slowed down by a factor of more than 100. This results in a marked prolongation of the sodium current across the nerve membrane during excitation, and this prolonged sodium current is directly responsible for the repetitive activity induced by allethrin (Vijverberg et al., 1983).

The effects of cismethrin on synaptic transmission in the frog neuromuscular junction, as reported by Evans (1976), are almost identical to those of allethrin, i.e., presynaptic repetitive firing, and no significant effects on transmitter release or on the subsynaptic membrane.

Interestingly, the action of these pyrethroids closely resembles that of the insecticide DDT in the peripheral nervous system of the frog. DDT also causes pronounced repetitive activity in sense organs, in sensory nerve fibres, and in motor nerve terminals, due to a prolongation of the transient increase in sodium permeability of the nerve membrane during excitation. Recently, it was demonstrated that allethrin and DDT have essentially the same effect on sodium channels in frog myelinated nerve membrane. Both compounds slow down the rate of closing of a fraction of the sodium channels that open on depolarization of the membrane (Van den Bercken et al., 1973, 1979; Vijverberg et al., 1982b).

In the electrophysiological experiments using giant axons of crayfish, the type I pyrethroids and DDT analogues retain sodium channels in a modified open state only intermittently, cause large depolarizing after-potentials, and evoke repetitive firing with minimal effect on the resting potential (Lund & Narahashi, 1983).

These results strongly suggest that permethrin and cismethrin, like allethrin, primarily affect the sodium channels in the nerve membrane and cause a prolongation of the transient increase in sodium permeability of the membrane during excitation.

The effects of pyrethroids on end-plate and muscle action potentials were studied in the pectoralis nerve-muscle preparation of the clawed frog (*Xenopus laevis*). Type I pyrethroids (allethrin, cismethrin, bioresmethrin, and 1R, *cis*-phenothrin) caused moderate presynaptic repetitive activity, resulting in the occurrence of multiple end-plate potentials (Ruigt & Van den Bercken, 1986).

### Pyrethroids with an α-cyano group on the 3-phenoxybenzyl alcohol (deltamethrin, cypermethrin, fenvalerate, and fenpropanate) (Type II: CS-syndrome)

The pyrethroids with an α-cyano group cause an intense repetitive activity in the lateral line organ in the form of long-lasting last for up to 1 min and contains thousands of impulses. The duration of the trains and the number of impulses per train increase markedly on lowering the temperature. Cypermethrin does not cause repetitive activity in myelinated nerve fibres. Instead, this pyrethroid causes a frequency-dependent depression of the nervous impulse, brought about by a progressive depolarization of the nerve membrane as a result of the summation of depolarizing after-potentials during train stimulation (Vijverberg & Van den Bercken, 1979; Vijverberg et al., 1983).

In the isolated node of Ranvier, cypermethrin, like allethrin, specifically affects the sodium channels of the nerve membrane and causes a long-lasting prolongation of the transient increase in sodium permeability during excitation, presumably by slowing down the closing of the activation gate of the sodium channel (Vijverberg & Van den Bercken, 1979; Vijverberg et al., 1983). The time constant of closing of the activation gate in the cypermethrin-affected channels is prolonged to more than 100 milliseconds. Apparently, the amplitude of the prolonged sodium current after cypermethrin is too small to induce repetitive activity in nerve fibres, but is sufficient to cause the long-lasting repetitive firing in the lateral-line sense organ.

These results suggest that α-cyano pyrethroids primarily affect the sodium channels in the nerve membrane and cause a long-lasting prolongation of the transient increase in sodium permeability of the membrane during excitation.

In the electrophysiological experiments using giant axons of crayfish, the Type II pyrethroids retain sodium channels in a modified continuous open state persistently, depolarize the membrane, and block the action potential without causing repetitive firing (Lund & Narahashi, 1983).

Diazepam, which facilitates GABA reaction, delayed the onset of action of deltamethrin and fenvalerate, but not permethrin and allethrin, in both the mouse and cockroach. Possible mechanisms of the Type II pyrethroid syndrome include action at the GABA receptor complex or a closely linked class of neuroreceptor (Gammon et al., 1982).

The Type II syndrome of intracerebrally administered pyrethroids closely approximates that of the convulsant picrotoxin (PTX). Deltamethrin inhibits the binding of [$^{3}$H]-dihydropicrotoxin to rat brain synaptic membranes, whereas the non-toxic R epimer of deltamethrin is inactive. These findings suggest a possible relation between the Type II pyrethroid action and the GABA receptor complex. The stereospecific correlation between the toxicity of Type II pyrethroids and their potency to inhibit the [$^{35}$S]-TBPS binding was established using a radioligand, [$^{35}$S]-*t*-butyl-bicyclophosphorothionate [$^{35}$S]-TBPS. Studies with 37 pyrethroids revealed an absolute correlation, without any false positive or negative, between mouse intracerebral toxicity and *in vitro* inhibition: all toxic cyano compounds including deltamethrin, 1R,*cis*-cypermethrin, 1R,*trans*-cypermethrin, and [2S, $\alpha$ S]-fenvalerate were inhibitors, but their non-toxic stereoisomers were not; non-cyano pyrethroids were much less potent or were inactive (Lawrence & Casida, 1983).

In the [$^{35}$S]-TBPS and [$^{3}$H]-Ro 5-4864 (a convulsant benzodiazepine radioligand) binding assay, the inhibitory potencies of pyrethroids were closely related to their mammalian toxicities. The most toxic pyrethroids of Type II were the most potent inhibitors of [$^{3}$H]-Ro 5-4864 specific binding to rat brain membranes. The [$^{3}$H]-dihydropicrotoxin and [$^{35}$S]-TBPS binding studies with pyrethroids strongly indicated that Type II effects of pyrethroids are mediated, at least in part, through an interaction with a GABA-regulated chloride ionophore-associated binding site. Moreover, studies with [$^{3}$H]-Ro 5-4864 support this hypothesis and, in addition, indicate that the pyrethroid-binding site may be very closely related to the convulsant benzodiazepine site of action (Lawrence et al., 1985).

The Type II pyrethroids (deltamethrin, 1R, *cis*-cypermethrin and [2S, $\alpha$S]-fenvalerate) increased the input resistance of crayfish claw opener muscle fibres bathed in GABA. In contrast, two non-insecticidal stereoisomers and Type I pyrethroids (permethrin, resmethrin, allethrin) were inactive. Therefore, cyanophenoxybenzyl pyrethroids appear to act on the GABA receptor-ionophore complex (Gammon & Casida, 1983).

The effects of pyrethroids on end-plate and muscle action potentials were studied in the pectoralis nerve-muscle preparation of the clawed frog (*Xenopus laevis*). Type II pyrethroids (cypermethrin and deltamethrin) induced trains of repetitive muscle action potentials without presynaptic repetitive activity. However, an intermediate group of pyrethroids (1R-permethrin, cyphenothrin, and fenvalerate) caused both types of effect. Thus, in muscle or nerve membrane the pyrethroid induced repetitive activities due to a prolongation of the sodium current. But no clear distinction was observed between non-cyano and α-cyano pyrethroids (Ruigt & Van den Bercken, 1986).

## Appraisal

In summary, the results strongly suggest that the primary target site of pyrethroid insecticides in the vertebrate nervous system is the sodium channel in the nerve membrane. Pyrethroids without an α-cyano group (allethrin, d-phenothrin, permethrin, and cismethrin) cause a moderate prolongation of the transient increase in sodium permeability of the nerve membrane during excitation. This results in relatively short trains of repetitive nerve impulses in sense organs, sensory (afferent) nerve fibres, and, in effect, nerve terminals. On the other hand, the α-cyano pyrethroids cause a long-lasting prolongation of the transient increase in sodium permeability of the nerve membrane during excitation. This results in long-lasting trains of repetitive impulses in sense organs and a frequency-dependent depression of the nerve impulse in nerve fibres. The difference in effects between permethrin and cypermethrin, which have identical molecular structures except for the presence of an α-cyano group on the phenoxybenzyl alcohol, indicates that it is this α-cyano group that is responsible for the long-lasting prolongation of the sodium permeability.

Since the mechanisms responsible for nerve impulse generation and conduction are basically the same throughout the entire nervous system, pyrethroids may also induce repetitive activity in various parts of the brain. The difference in symptoms of poisoning by α-cyano pyrethroids, compared with the classical pyrethroids, is not necessarily due to an exclusive central site of action.

It may be related to the long-lasting repetitive activity in sense organs and possibly in other parts of the nervous system, which, in a more advance state of poisoning, may be accompanied by a frequency-dependent depression of the nervous impulse.

Pyrethroids also cause pronounced repetitive activity and a prolongation of the transient increase in sodium permeability of the nerve membrane in insects and other invertebrates. Available information indicates that the sodium channel in the nerve membrane is also the most important target site of pyrethroids in the invertebrate nervous system (Wouters & Van den Bercken, 1978; WHO, 1979).

Because of the universal character of the processes underlying nerve excitability, the action of pyrethroids should not be considered restricted to particular animal species, or to a certain region of the nervous system. Although it has been established that sense organs and nerve endings are the most vulnerable to the action of pyrethroids, the ultimate lesion that causes death will depend on the animal species, environmental conditions, and on the chemical structure and physical characteristics of the pyrethroid molecule (Vijverberg & Van den Bercken, 1982).

# 1. RESUME ET EVALUATION, CONCLUSIONS ET RECOMMANDATIONS

## 1.1 Résumé et évaluation

### 1.1.1 *Identité, propriétés physiques et chimiques, méthodes d'analyse*

La deltaméthrine a été synthétisée en 1974 et commercialisée pour la première fois en 1977. Sur le plan chimique, c'est un ester de l'analogue dibromé de l'acide chrysanthémique (acide diméthyl-2,2(dimbromo-2,2 vinyl)-3 cyclopropanecarboxylique) ($Br_2CA$) et de l'alcool α-cyano-phénoxy-3 benzylique; plus précisément, c'est l'isomère [1R,*cis*;α S] parmi les huit stéréo-isomères que compte cet ester.

La deltaméthrine de qualité technique se présente sous la forme d'une poudre blanche inodore dont le point de fusion est de 98–101 °C et qui contient plus de 98% de deltaméthrine. Sa tension de vapeur est de $2{,}0 \times 10^{6}$ Pa à 25 °C; autrement dit, elle n'est pratiquement pas volatile. Insoluble dans l'eau, elle est en revanche soluble dans des solvants organiques tels que l'acétone, la cyclohexanone et le xylène. Elle est stable à la lumière, à la chaleur et à l'air, mais instable en milieu alcalin.

Pour doser les résidus et analyser des échantillons prélevés dans l'environnement, on procède à une extraction par solvant au moyen d'un mélange *n*-hexane/acétone, à un partage entre le *n*-hexane, l'acétone et l'eau, suivi d'une purification par chromatographie sur colonne de gel de silice, le dosage final s'effectuant par chromatographie en phase gazeuse avec détection par capture d'électrons. La concentration minimale décelable par cette méthode est de 0,01 mg/kg, voire moins. L'analyse des produits s'effectue par chromatographie en phase liquide à haute performance avec détecteur UV.

### 1.1.2 *Production et usage*

En 1987, la consommation mondiale de deltaméthrine était d'environ 250 tonnes. On l'utilise essentiellement pour traiter le coton (45% de la consommation) ainsi que pour les cultures telles que le café, le maïs, les céréales, les fruits, les légumes, le houblon et les produits stockés. On l'utilise aussi pour l'hygiène des animaux, la lutte contre les vecteurs ainsi qu'à des fins de santé publique. On l'applique soit seule, soit associée à d'autres pesticides en formulations telles que concentrés émulsionnables, concentrés pour pulvérisation à très bas volume, poudres mouillables, concentrés pour suspension, poudres pour poudrage, etc.

### 1.1.3 Exposition humaine

L'exposition de la population dans son ensemble provient principalement de la présence de résidus alimentaires mais peut également résulter de son utilisation en santé publique. Sur les récoltes correctement traitées, le taux de résidus est généralement très faible sauf lorsque le traitement a eu lieu après la récolte. La FAO et l'OMS ont passé en revue de nombreuses données sur ces questions.

L'exposition de la population dans son ensemble est vraisemblablement très faible, mais on manque de données effectives découlant d'études sur la ration alimentaire totale.

### 1.1.4 Exposition et destinée dans l'environnement

En exposant à la lumière solaire une fine pellicule de deltaméthrine [1R, *cis*; α S] marquée au $C^{14}$ au niveau de la fonction acide, de la fonction alcool ou du groupe cyano, pendant 4 à 8 heures, on a constaté que 70 % du produit était transformé en isomères [1R, *trans* α S] et [1S, *trans* α S] par isomérisation *cis/trans*, accompagnés des produits de clivage de l'ester, en particulier l'acide diméthyl-2,2(dibromovinyl-2,2)-3 cyclopropane-carboxylique et l'alcool α-cyano-phénoxy-3 benzylique.

La deltaméthrine présente sur des plants de coton en serre se dégrade avec une demi-vie initiale de 1,1 semaine, le taux de dégradation étant de 90 % au bout de 4,5 semaines.

Les principaux métabolites consistent en $Br_2CA$ libre et conjugué, en *trans*-hydroxyméthyl-$Br_2CA$ et en acide (hydroxy-4 phénoxy)-3 benzoïque résultant du clivage de l'ester, d'une oxydation et d'une conjugaison.

Après avoir fait incuber de deltaméthrine dans du sable et du terreau à 28 °C dans les conditions du laboratoire, on en a récupéré respectivement 52 % et 74 %, huit semaines après ce traitement.

La deltaméthrine ne se déplace pas dans l'environnement du fait qu'elle est fortement adsorbée sur les particules, qu'elle est insoluble dans l'eau et qu'elle est appliquée à très faibles doses.

On ne dispose pas de données sur les concentrations effectives dans l'environnement, mais compte tenu des modalités actuelles d'utilisation et pour peu que l'insecticide soit utilisé normalement, l'exposition environnementale devrait être très faible. La deltaméthrine se dégrade rapidement en produits moins toxiques.

### 1.1.5 *Absorption, métabolisme et excrétion*

Administrée par voie orale, la deltraméthrine est facilement absorbée; l'absorption est moindre par la voie percutanée encore que sa vitesse dépende fortement du véhicule ou du solvant utilisé. Une fois absorbée, la deltaméthrine est rapidement métabolisée et excrétée.

On a administré à des rats par voie orale, à raison de 0,64 à 1,60 mg/kg, de la deltaméthrine marquée au carbone-14 au niveau des fonctions acide, alcool et nitrile; le radio-carbone provenant de la fraction acide et de la fraction alcoolique a été complètement éliminé en l'espace de 2 à 4 jours. Les taux de résidus tissulaires étaient généralement faibles sauf dans les graisses où ils étaient un peu plus élevés. Cependant, le reste nitrile a été excrété plus lentement, le taux global de récupération étant de 79 % en huit jours. Les principales réactions métaboliques étaient l'oxydation (au niveau du méthyl-*trans*, du cycle cyclopropane et des positions 2', 4' et 5' du reste alcoolique), le clivage de l'ester et la conversion du nitrile en thiocyanate. Les acides carboxyliques et les phénols résultants étaient conjugués à l'acide sulfurique, à la glycine et à l'acide glucuronique.

Après avoir administré par voie orale à des souris de la deltaméthrine marquée au $^{14}C$ au niveau des fonctions acide, alcool et nitrile à raison de 1,7 et 4,4 mg/kg, on a constaté que l'excrétion du radiocarbone s'effectuait rapidement sauf dans le cas du reste nitrile. Les principales réactions métaboliques étaient en général analogues chez les souris et chez les rats.

Chez les vaches et la volaille, les voies de dégradation sont tout à fait analogues à celles des rongeurs.

### 1.1.6 *Effets sur les êtres vivants dans leur milieu naturel*

La deltaméthrine est extrêmement toxique pour les poissons, la $CL_{50}$ à 96 heures allant de 0,4 à 2,0 µg/litre. Elle est également très toxique pour les invertébrés aquatiques; pour la daphnie, la $CL_{50}$ à 48 heures est de 5 µg/litre. Toutefois des études approfondies sur des étangs expérimentaux ainsi que les résultats de l'utilisation en plein champ ont montré que cette forte toxicité potentielle était inopérante. On a observé sur le terrain une certaine mortalité parmi les invertébrés aquatiques mais les populations se reconstituent généralement assez vite.

Pour les oiseaux, la toxicité de la deltaméthrine est très faible, les valeurs de la $DL_{50}$ pour une dose unique par voie orale étant supérieure à 1000 mg/kg. Au laboratoire, la deltaméthrine est très toxique pour les abeilles, avec une $DL_{50}$ de contact de 0,051 µg/abeille. Les essais en situation réelle et l'expérience acquise dans l'utilisation effective du produit ont montré que les formulations de deltaméthrine exerçaient une action répulsive, ce qui signifie qu'en pratique le danger pour les abeilles est très réduit.

### 1.1.7 *Effets sur les animaux d'expérience et systemes d'épreuve in vitro*

Dans un véhicule non aqueux, la deltaméthrine présente une toxicité aiguë par voie orale forte à modérée avec des $DL_{50}$ de 19 à 34mg/kg chez la souris et de 39 à 139 mg/kg chez le rat. Toutefois, en suspension dans l'eau, la toxicité est bien moindre, les valeurs de la $DL_{50}$ dépassant 5000 mg/kg chez le rat. La deltaméthrine est un pyréthroide du Type II. Les signes cliniques d'intoxication consistent en tremblements, salivation et convulsions. L'intoxication est rapide et chez les survivants, les signes disparaissent en quelques jours. L'électro-encéphalogramme présente des décharges pointes-ondes généralisées qui précèdent la choréo-athétose.

Une seule application de deltaméthrine technique n'a pas produit d'effets irritants sur la peau intacte ou abrasée du lapin. Toutefois elle a produit des effets irritants passagers au niveau de l'oeil avec ou sans rinçage. La deltaméthrine n'a pas d'effet sensibilisateur cutané chez le cobaye.

En administrant à des rats par gavage de la deltaméthrine à des doses quotidiennes allant jusqu'à 10 mg/kg de poids corporel pendant 13 semaines, on a provoqué chez ces animaux une hyperexcitabilité qui se manifestait au bout de six semaines chez les mâles recevant la dose la plus forte. Aux doses de 2,5 et 10 mg/kg, le gain de poids a été plus faible chez les mâles.

Chez des chiens beagle qui avaient reçu par voie orale de la deltaméthrine en doses quotidiennes allant jusqu'à 10 mg/kg de poids corporel pendant 13 semaines, on a observé divers symptômes liés à cette substance, tels que des vomissements, des tremblements, de la salivation et un affaiblissement du réflexe pharyngé, du réflexe rotulien et du réflexe de flexion. Lors d'une étude d'alimentation de deux ans sur des chiens, on a constaté que la dose sans effet observable se situait à 1 mg/kg de poids corporel par jour (dose la plus forte expérimentée).

L'administration de deltraméthrine à des souris à des doses atteignant 100 mg/kg de nourriture pendant 24 mois n'a pas modifié l'incidence des tumeurs. La dose sans effet observé relative à la toxicité générale était de 100 mg/kg de nourriture.

Chez des rats à qui l'on avait administré de la deltaméthrine en doses allant jusqu'à 50 mg/kg de nourriture pendant deux ans, on n'a observé aucune tumeur attribuable à cette substance. La dose sans effet observé relative à la toxicité générale était de 5 mg/kg de nourriture.

La deltaméthrine ne s'est pas révélée mutagène dans divers systèmes d'épreuve *in vivo* et *in vitro*; notamment la réparation de l'ADN, la mutation génique, les aberrations chromosomiques, l'échange entre chromatides-soeurs, la formation de micronoyaux et la létalité dominante.

Des études de tératogénicité ont été effectuées chez des rates et des souris gravides à qui l'on administrait par voie orale des doses quotidiennes de deltaméthrine allant jusqu'à 1000 mg/kg pendant la phase principale de l'organogénèse. On n'a constaté aucun effet tératogène ni altération de la fonction de reproduction chez ces rates et ces souris, si ce n'est une réduction, liée à la dose, dans le poids moyen des foetus chez les souris et un léger retard d'ossification chez les rats.

Des lapines gravides ont reçu au sixième et dix-neuvième jours de leur grossesse des doses quotidiennes de deltaméthrine allant jusqu'à 16 mg/kg. A la dose la plus forte, on a noté une réduction du poids moyen des foetus. Aucun effet tératogène n'a été observé chez les lapins.

Après administration de deltaméthrine à des rats à des doses allant jusqu'à 5 mg/kg de nourriture, dans le but d'effectuer une étude de reproduction sur trois générations et deux portées, on a constaté l'absence totale de tout effet.

Il existe certains indices selon lesquels l'association de deltaméthrine à certains composés organophosphorés pourrait conduire à une potentialisation de la toxicité de ces produits.

### 1.1.8 *Effets sur l'homme*

La deltaméthrine peut provoquer certaines sensations cutanées chez des travailleurs exposés. Plusieurs cas d'intoxication professionnelle non mortelle ont été signalés qui étaient dus à l'inobservation des mesures de sécurité. Un engourdissement, un prurit, des fourmillements et une sensation de brûlure de la peau ainsi que des vertiges sont des symptômes fréquemment signalés. On a décrit occasionnellement un érythème papulaire ou une couperose à caractère passager. La plupart de ces symptômes sont passagers et disparaissent en cinq à sept jours. Aucun effet indésirable à long terme n'a été signalé. On a décrit trois cas d'empoisonnement non mortel par la deltaméthrine à la suite de l'ingestion de plusieurs grammes de ce produit.

## 1.2 Conclusions

*Population générale*: l'exposition de la population générale à la deltaméthrine est vraisemblablement très faible et ce produit, lorsqu'il est utilisé conformément aux recommandations, ne présente probablement aucun risque.

*Exposition professionnelle*: moyennant de bonnes méthodes de travail et l'application de mesures d'hygiène et de sécurité, la deltaméthrine ne devrait pas présenter de danger pour les personnes qui y sont exposées de par leur profession.

*Environnement*: Utilisée aux doses recommandées, il est improbable que la deltaméthrine ou ses produits de dégradation s'accumulent au point d'avoir des effets nocifs sur l'environnement. Au laboratoire, la deltaméthrine est très toxique pour les poissons, les arthropodes aquatiques et les abeilles. Toutefois, sur le terrain, il est peu probable que le produit ait des effets nocifs s'il est utilisé conformément aux recommandations.

## 1.3 Recommandations

Bien que les teneurs dans les aliments soient très faibles lorsque la deltaméthrine est utilisée conformément aux recommandations, il est souhaitable de s'en assurer en soumettant la deltaméthrine à une surveillance.

La deltaméthrine est utilisée depuis de nombreuses années et l'on signale un certain nombre de cas d'intoxications non mortelles ainsi que des effets passagers par suite d'exposition professionnelle. Il est souhaitable que l'exposition humaine continue d'être surveillée.

# 1. RESUMEN Y EVALUACION, CONCLUSIONES Y RECOMENDACIONES

## 1.1 Resumen y evaluación

### *1.1.1 Identidad, propiedades físicas y químicas, métodos de análisis*

La deltametrina fue sintetizada en 1974 y se comercializó por primera vez en 1977. Químicamente, es el isómero [1R,*cis*; S] de 8 ésteres estereoisoméricos del análogo dibromo del ácido crisantémico, ácido 2,2-dimetil-3-(2,2-dibromovinil) ciclopropanocarboxílico ($Br_2CA$) con alcohol α-ciano-3-fenoxibencílico.

La deltametrina de calidad técnica es un polvo blanco inodoro con un punto de fusión de 98–101 °C y contiene más del 98% del material. La presión del vapor es $2{,}0 \times 10^{-6}$ Pa a 25 °C y es prácticamente no volátil. Es insoluble en agua, pero soluble en disolventes orgánicos como la acetona, la ciclohexanona y el xileno. Es estable a la luz, el calor y el aire, pero inestable en medios alcalinos.

La determinación de la presencia de residuos y el análisis de muestras ambientales se efectuaron por extracción con los disolventes *n*-hexano/acetona, partición con *n*-hexano/acetona/agua, absorción con un cromatógrafo de columna de gel de sílice y determinación con un cromatógrafo de fase gaseosa equipado con un detector de captura de electrones con una concentración mínima detectable de 0,01 mg/kg o menos. Para el análisis de productos se utiliza la cromatografía de fase líquida de alto rendimiento con un detector de rayos UV.

### *1.1.2 Producción y empleo*

El consumo mundial de deltametrina era de 250 toneladas aproximadamente en 1987. La deltametrina se utiliza sobre todo en el algodón (45% del consumo), en cultivos como el café, el maíz, los cereales, la fruta, las hortalizas y el lúpulo, y en productos almacenados. Se emplea también en higiene animal, en la lucha contra los vectores y en salud pública. Se fabrica como solución concentrada emulsionable, solución concentrada de pequeñísimo volumen, polvo humectable, solución concentrada en suspensión y polvo para utilización en seco, sola o en combinación con otros plaguicidas.

### 1.1.3 *Exposición humana*

La exposición de la población en general a la deltametrina procede principalmente de residuos en la dieta, pero puede resultar también de su empleo en salud pública. En los cultivos tratados de acuerdo con buenas prácticas agrícolas, las concentraciones residuales son por lo general muy bajas, excepto en caso de tratamiento después de la recolección. La FAO y la OMS han examinado abundantes datos al respecto.

Se cree que la exposición de la población en general es muy baja, pero no se dispone de datos en forma de estudios de dietas totales.

### 1.1.4 *Exposición ambiental y evolución*

Cuando la deltametrina-[1R,*cis;* α S] *marcada con* $C^{14}$-(compuesto irradiado ácido, alcohol o ciano) se expuso a la luz del sol en forma de una película fina durante 4 a 8 horas, el 70% se transformó por isomerización-*cis*/*trans* produciendo los isómeros [1R,*trans*; α S] y [1S,*trans*; α S], junto con productos de la escisión de los ésteres, entre ellos $Br_2CA$ y alcohol α-ciano-3-fenoxibencílico.

La deltametrina se degradó en las plantas de algodón, en condiciones de invernadero, con una vida media inicial de 1,1 semanas, y el tiempo necesario para una pérdida del 90% fue de 4,6 semanas.

Los principales metabolitos fueron $Br_2CA$ libre y combinado, *trans*-hidroximetil-$Br_2CA$ y ácido 3-(4-hidroxifenoxi)benzoico, formados por la escisión, la oxidación y la combinación de los ésteres.

La deltametrina se incubó en arena y mantillo orgánico a 28 °C en condiciones de laboratorio. Ocho semanas después del tratamiento, se recuperó de la arena y del mantillo orgánico alrededor del 52% y el 74%, respectivamente, de la deltametrina aplicada.

La deltametrina no es móvil en el medio debido a su fuerte adsorción en las partículas, su insolubilidad en el agua y sus tasas muy bajas de aplicación.

No se dispone de datos sobre las concentraciones existentes en el medio pero, dadas las modalidades actuales de uso y en condiciones normales, es de esperar que la exposición ambiental sea muy baja. Se degrada rápidamente, convirtiéndose en productos menos tóxicos.

### 1.1.5 Ingestion, metabolismo y excreción

La deltametrina se absorbe fácilmente por vía oral y con menor facilidad por la piel, pero la tasa de absorción depende considerablemente del portador o disolvente. La deltametrina absorbida se metaboliza y se excreta fácilmente.

En la administración por vía oral a ratas de deltametrina marcada con $C^{14}$-(compuesto irradiado ácido, alcohol o ciano), a tasas de 0,64-1,60 mg/kg, el radiocarbono de las partes ácido y alcohol se eliminó casi por completo en 2-4 días. Las concentraciones residuales en los tejidos fueron por lo general muy bajas, excepto en la grasa, en donde fueron ligeramente más altas. Sin embargo, la parte ciano se excretó más lentamente, con una recuperación total del 79% en 8 días. Las principales reacciones metabólicas fueron oxidación (en el *trans*-metilo del anillo de ciclopropano y en las posiciones 2'-, 4'-, y 5 de la parte alcohol), escisión de ésteres y conversión de la parte ciano en tiocianato. Los ácidos carboxílicos y fenoles resultantes se combinaron con ácido sulfúrico, glicocola y ácido glucurónico.

Cuando se administró a ratones $C^{14}$-(compuesto irradiado ácido, alcohol o ciano)-deltametrina por vía oral, a tasas de 1,7–4,4 mg/kg, la excreción del radiocarbono fue rápida y casi total, excepto en la parte ciano. Las principales reacciones metabólicas observadas en los ratones fueron en general semejantes a las observadas en las ratas.

En el ganado vacuno y las aves de corral, las vías de degradación son muy similares a las observadas en los roedores.

### 1.1.6 Efectos en los organismos presentes en el medio

La deltametrina es muy tóxica para los peces, ya que la $CL_{50}$ en 96 horas oscila entre 0,4 y 2,0 µg/litro. Es también muy tóxica para los invertebrados acuáticos: la $CL_{50}$ en 48 horas para *Daphnia* es de 5 µg/litro. Sin embargo, extensos estudios realizados en estanques experimentales y el empleo sobre el terreno han demostrado que esa elevada toxicidad potencial no llega a concretarse. En la práctica hay algunas muertes de invertebrados acuáticos que, por lo general, se compensan con rapidez.

La toxicidad de la deltametrina en las aves es muy baja, con valores de la $DL_{50}$ superiores a 1000 mg/kg cuando se administra una sola dosis por vía oral. En condiciones de laboratorio, la deltametrina es muy tóxica para las abejas, con una $DL_{50}$ por contacto de 0,051 µg/abeja. Los ensayos sobre el terreno y el empleo no experimental han demostrado que los preparados de deltametrina tienen una acción repelente, lo cual quiere decir que, en la práctica, el riesgo para las abejas es escaso.

### 1.1.7 Efectos en animales experimentales y en sistemas de pruebas in vitro

En un vehículo no acuoso, la toxicidad de la deltametrina administrada por vía oral en forma aguda va de alta a moderada, con $DL_{50}$ de 19 a 34 mg/kg (ratones) y de 31 a 139 mg/kg (ratas). Sin embargo, cuando la deltametrina está en suspensión en agua, su toxicidad es mucho menor con $DL_{50}$ superiores a 5000 mg/kg (ratas). La deltametrina es un piretroide de tipo II; los signos clínicos comprenden temblor, salivación y convulsiones. La intoxicación se presenta rápidamente y, en los supervivientes, los signos desaparecen en unos días. El electroencefalograma muestra descargas generalizadas en picos y ondas, seguidas de coreoatetosis.

Aplicaciones únicas de deltametrina técnica no tuvieron ningún efecto irritante en la piel, intacta o con abrasiones, de conejos. Sin embargo, se observaron efectos irritantes transitorios en los ojos de conejos, con y sin lavado. La deltametrina no actuó como sensibilizante dérmico en cobayas.

En ratas a las que se administró deltametrina con sonda, en dosis de hasta 10,0 mg/kg de peso corporal diarios durante 13 semanas, a las 6 semanas se observó hiperexcitabilidad en los machos que habían recibido la dosis más alta. El aumento del peso corporal en los machos fue menor con dosis de 2,5 y 10 mg/kg.

En perros de la raza beagle a los que se administró por vía oral deltametrina en dosis de hasta 10 mg/kg de peso corporal diarios durante 13 semanas, se observaron varios síntomas relacionados con el compuesto, como vómitos, temblor, salivación y reflejos faríngeo, patelar y flexor deprimidos. En un estudio de alimentación en perros, de dos años de duración, la dosis desprovista de efectos fue de 1 mg/kg de peso corporal diario (dosis más alta estudiada).

En ratones a los que se administró deltametrina en dosis de hasta 100 mg/kg de alimentos durante 24 meses, no resultó afectada la incidencia de tumores. En cuanto a la toxicidad general, la dosis desprovista de efectos fue de 100 mg/kg de alimentos.

En ratas a las que se administró deltametrina a niveles de hasta 50 mg/kg de alimentos durante dos años, no se observaron tumores relacionados con el compuesto. La concentración desprovista de efectos de la toxicidad general fue de 50 mg/kg de alimentos.

No se observaron efectos mutagénicos de la deltametrina en una multitud de sistemas de pruebas *in vivo* e *in vitro*, incluidos: reparación del ADN, mutación génica, aberración cromosómica, intercambio de cromátidas hermanas, formación de micronúcleos y genes letales dominantes.

Se realizaron estudios teratológicos con ratas y ratonas preñadas, administrando deltametrina por vía oral en dosis de hasta 10 mg/kg diarias durante el periodo de mayor organogénesis. No se observaron efectos teratogénicos ni reproductivos en las ratas ni en las ratonas, excepto una disminución, relacionada con la dosis, del peso fetal medio en el estudio con ratonas y una osificación ligeramente retrasada en el estudio con ratas.

Se administró a conejas deltametrina en dosis de hasta 16 mg/kg diarios entre los días 6 y 19 del embarazo. Con la dosis más alta, se registró una disminución del peso fetal medio. No se observaron efectos teratogénicos.

Se administró a ratas deltametrina en dosis de hasta 50 mg/kg de alimentos en un estudio sobre reproducción con tres generaciones y dos camadas, sin que se observaran efectos sobre la reproducción.

Hay indicios de que la toxicidad puede potenciarse cuando la deltametrina se combina con algunos compuestos organofosforados.

### 1.1.8 *Efectos en los seres humanos*

La deltametrina puede provocar sensaciones cutáneas en los trabajadores expuestos. Se han notificado varios casos de intoxicación no mortal debidos a exposición ocupacional por no respetar las precauciones de seguridad. Son síntomas frecuentemente mencionados adormecimiento, picor, hormigueo y quemazón de la piel, y vértigo. En ocasiones se ha descrito un eritema papular o maculoso. La mayor parte de esos síntomas son temporales y desaparecen en 5 ó 7 días. No se han comunicado efectos negativos a largo plazo. Se han descrito tres casos no mortales de intoxicación por deltametrina tras la ingestión de varios gramos del producto.

## 1.2 Conclusiones

*Población en general*: No es probable que la exposición de la población en general a la deltametrina, que se cree muy baja, represente un riesgo en las condiciones de empleo recomendadas.

*Exposición ocupacional*: Si se aplican buenas prácticas laborales, medidas de higiene y precauciones de seguridad, no es probable que la deltametrina represente un riesgo para las personas ocupacionalmente expuestas a ella.

*Medio ambiente*: Es improbable que la deltametrina o los productos de su degradación alcancen niveles que puedan tener efectos negativos en el medio con las tasas de aplicación recomendadas. En condiciones de laboratorio, la deltametrina es muy tóxica para los peces, los artrópodos acuáticos y las abejas. No obstante, en la práctica, no es probable que haya efectos perjudiciales duraderos con las condiciones de empleo recomendadas.

## 1.3 Recomendaciones

Aunque se cree que con el uso recomendado las concentraciones en la dieta son muy bajas, debe considerarse la conveniencia de confirmarlo incluyendo la deltametrina en estudios de vigilancia.

La deltametrina se utiliza desde hace muchos años y se han notificado varios casos de intoxicación no mortal y efectos transitorios debidos a exposición ocupacional. Debe mantenerse la observación de la exposición humana.